THE BACKCOUNTRY CLASSROOM

Lesson Plans for Teaching in the Wilderness

by
Bruce F. Bonney
And
Jack K. Drury

, Inc.
.ilville, IN

The Backcountry Classroom
Lesson Plans for Teaching in the Wilderness

Copyright © 1992 by
The Wilderness Education Association
20 Winona Avenue, Box 89
Saranac Lake, New York 12983
(518) 891-2915 Ext 254

Bruce F. Bonney
Social Studies Teacher
Morrisville-Eaton Central School
Morrisville, NY

Jack K. Drury
Associate Professor and Director
Wilderness Recreation Leadership Program
North Country Community College
Saranac Lake, NY

Published by:
ICS Books, Inc.
One Tower Plaza
107 E. 89th Avenue
Merrillville, IN 46410
800/541-7323

The Backcountry Classroom was partially funded by grants from the Adirondack North Country Association and International Paper Company

Printed in the U.S.A.

The Backcountry Classroom was partially funded by grants from the Adirondack North Country Association and International Paper Company Foundation

Cover photo by Mark Kurtz

Library of Congress Cataloging-in Publication Data

Bonney, Bruce F.
     The backcountry classroom lesson plans for teaching in the
wilderness / by Bruce F. Bonney and Jack K. Drury.
          p.   cm.
     Includes index.
     ISBN 0-934802-18-1
     1. Outdoor education.   I. Drury, Jack K.   II. Title.
LB1047.B55   1992
371.3'8--dc20   92-26151
                                                      CIP

Dedication

To Jack: For showing the way…
                    B.F.B

To Carmen: For assisting me in the
     pursuit of my dreams.

To Eli and Dustin: May they reap the
     rewards the wilderness has to
     offer.
                    J.K.D.

In Appreciation

To Kim Massari for turning our work into
     something we can be proud of.

Contents

FOOD PREPARATION

NAVIGATION

SAFETY

Acknowledgments

Many people have assisted in the creation of this manual. We would like to especially thank the authors who wrote specific lesson plans: Chris Cashel, Michael Kudish, Brian McDonnell, and Mary Vance as well as Larry Alonso and Glenn Clark who assisted in the development of a number of the lesson plans. In addition we would like to recognize WEA Board members Paul Petzoldt, David Cockrell, Mitchell Sakofs, Bill Forgey, Sandy Bridges, Bill Shiner, and Frank Lupton for their assistance in providing input on various lesson plans. WEA Executive Director Mark Wagstaff and office personnel Kathy Jurczynski, Duane Gould, and Helena Gladke also provided help in many ways in the development of this project. Rory Gillespie of Better Image Graphics contributed many hours designing and laying out the draft copy. We are extremely grateful to Kim Massari for editing and creating the final layout of this book, Dr. Jim Glover for proofreading the final draft, Christina Newkirk for helping with design, and Mark Kurtz for his time photographing the cover.

North Country Community College played an instrumental role in the creation of this book. Former College President David Petty was an unqualified supporter of WEA whose premature death was a tragic loss for both North Country Community College and WEA. Academic Dean Gail Rogers Rice and Division Chair Ross Dailey provided support in numerous ways. Brian Allen of the Printing Department helped turn our work into reality, Meg Bernstein provided illustrations, and Richard Rice offered computer assistance.

WEA Curriculum Advisory Board members David Bates, Paul Brown, Stan Bush, Kelly Cain, Chris Cashel, Kent Clement, Dee Edelman, Alan Ewert, Doug Fitzgerald, John Gamble, Dan Garvey, Lewis Glenn, Cliff Jacobson, Bunny Johns, Bjorn Kjellstrom, Michael Moniz, Walt Meyers, Maurice Phipps, Edward Raiola, Michael Selby, and Buck Tilton provided invaluable input in their careful review of our work as did Paul Smith's College faculty Dave Nettles and Ruth Smith, and Peter Biddle of North Country Community College.

We would like to give special recognition to North Country Community College Wilderness Recreation Leadership instructors and the many students who were the primary guinea pigs as we developed and experimented with these lesson plans.

Introduction

"When we know what we are about,
we are better at being about it."

Wilderness education pioneer Paul Petzoldt relates a story recalling his first harrowing ascent of the Grand Teton in Wyoming in 1924. Barely surviving the climb, Paul remarks in *The New Wilderness Handbook* that he and his companion "had succeeded through sheer guts and luck. We were improperly dressed, had insufficient food, and inadequate equipment, knew nothing of snow and ice techniques, and very little about rock climbing." Sobered by the experience, Petzoldt concluded that if he "wanted to live to be an old mountaineer, I could not take chances and be so uninformed about such dangerous activities. It was then that I began to study mountaineering skills, psychology, judgment, and conservation..."

Paul's quest to develop his own base of backcountry experience and expertise soon led him to reflect upon the appalling lack of skills and judgment that he observed among many wilderness users. As the popularity of wilderness recreational use rose during the late 1950s and 1960s, he was alarmed by the increase of reported injury and death among travelers in the backcountry. Equally troubling was the obvious damage that was done to the natural environment wherever unskilled or irresponsible recreationists passed.

By the mid 1960s, Paul was convinced that the survival of the American wilderness and the safety of those seeking to enjoy it required a massive effort at public education. But how could this be done? What should be taught? Who would teach it?

The struggle to answer these and other fundamental questions led Petzoldt and other outdoor professionals to organize and focus their efforts, and in 1977, Paul, in conjunction with Dr. Frank Lupton, Dr. Bob Christie, and Charles Gregory, founded the Wilderness Education Association (WEA). These founders were intent upon developing an educational organization which would train outdoor leaders in the skills and good judgment necessary to lead and teach the public in the proper use of wilderness areas. Inspired by Petzoldt's vision, the WEA was created to "promote the professionalization of outdoor leadership and to thereby improve the safety of outdoor trips and enhance the conservation of the wild outdoors."

It has now been fifteen years since the birth of the WEA. These years have seen hundreds of students and scores of instructors set out on wilderness expeditions in search of educational experiences. By living through and reflecting on these experiences, they have amassed an impressive body of knowledge. Their observations include suggestions about what does and does not work in the backcountry, what steps need to be followed to ensure quality decision making, and what qualities seem to be associated with good leadership. As with any core of knowledge, these ideas are subject to change as new insights and information are added to the collective consciousness.

A companion volume to this book, *The Wilderness Educator: The Wilderness Education Association's Curriculum Guide*, is the WEA's attempt to summarize the complete body of knowledge now deemed essential for WEA instructors. In the classroom or in the field, it serves as a reference for instructors who are expected to be masters of many trades as they lead students through the 28-35 day educational expeditions which are the backbone of the WEA training program. The book includes eight chapters which explore complex or poorly understood aspects of the WEA curriculum, and suggests references for more basic materials.

The Backcountry Classroom is designed to help instructors and students master and teach the WEA curriculum while in the field. To encourage its practical use, the book is formatted in self-contained lesson plans. Each lesson describes the overall goal, the specific objectives, the body of knowledge, and the materials necessary for teaching about a specific topic within the WEA curriculum. Included in each plan are suggestions for the timing of the lesson during the expedition and some teaching methods that we have used successfully.

We hope that *The Backcountry Classroom* will be carried in your pack or duffle and used by instructors and students in the field. During the five years it has taken to compile these plans, they have served as a handy reference for information, an outline for portions of a lecture or demonstration, a handout for class discussion, a reading for students preparing their own classes, and once (after five days of constant downpour) as a fire starter of last resort.

These lesson plans are designed to be part of an expedition's mobile library. The table of contents is arranged alphabetically so that instructors and students can readily find topics of interest. The table of contents is intentionally not designed to suggest a specific order of subject presentation because we encourage each instructor to exercise his or her own best judgment in this regard. The reader should also note that while we include specific teaching suggestions at the end of each plan, we have sprinkled comments or useful observations within the text of the lesson plan as well. These comments are offset with *italics* to distinguish them from the main body of information.

While these plans are very useful, they are not intended to function like recipes in some wilderness education cookbook. A novice should not sit in the comfort of his or her living room, read this volume, and then trek off into the deep woods confident in the illusion that she or he is now adequately prepared for backcountry travel. The information and suggestions contained herein are no substitute for the good judgment that comes from proper instruction and first-hand experience in backcountry living. As with many of life's endeavors, reading about wilderness recreation is no educational substitute for experiencing it.

Finally, it is important to note that *The Backcountry Classroom* is not inscribed upon tablets of stone. This is of both practical and symbolic importance; we wish to stress that these plans are organic in nature. Every time we use them we find some element, large or small, which could be changed or improved. This is completely in keeping with the WEA philosophy. The entire approach of the WEA is predicated upon the belief that "immutable rules are tools for fools." Just as with our students and instructors, we ask that you apply your best judgment in using these lesson plans. We urge that you approach this guide as an empiricist. If the information contained within proves accurate and our teaching suggestions work—great! If you believe that there are significant errors or omissions, by all means alter the lesson to fit your needs and please pass your thoughts on to us. We constantly examine our ideas through the hard lens of life experience. We welcome any observation which clarifies our vision.

Saranac Lake, NY
1992

1. Bathing and Washing

I. **GOAL:** To have participants bathe and wash clothes with minimum impact on the water sources and surrounding environment.

II. **OBJECTIVES:**
A. Participants will be able to bathe with minimal impact on the water sources and the surrounding environment.
B. Participants will be able to wash clothes with minimal impact on the water sources and the surrounding environment.
C. Participants will understand why washing with soap in lakes and streams is harmful to the environment both physically and aesthetically.
D. Participants will understand the importance of bathing and washing regularly in the outdoors.

III. **CONTENT:**
A. **Bathing and Washing —Why a Special Approach?**
Few will argue that water sources need protecting, but many do not realize or stop to think of the physical and aesthetic impact of washing in a water source.
1. **Physical impacts**
Most people are familiar with biodegradable soaps versus non-biodegradable soaps, but what are their impacts? Whether a soap is biodegradable or not, it can have a negative impact on the environment. The chemicals which make up soaps can be broken into two general categories – those which are nutrients and those which are toxic to plants and animals. One consequence of introducing soaps into the water ecosystem is called cultural eutrophication.

© 1992
The Wilderness Education Association
P.O. Box 89
Saranac Lake, New York 12983
(518) 891-2915 ext. 254

1

a.   **Cultural eutrophication**
Occurs in an aquatic environment in which the amounts of nutrients are abnormally high. It causes rapid growth of plant life which eventually reaches a point where the plant life blocks the sunlight. Without sunlight the plants cannot carry out photosynthesis and they die. When the plants die they consume oxygen and this loss of oxygen results in the death of many species, essentially by suffocation (Vivian, 1983). It is unknown what role wilderness users contribute to this phenomenon, but every effort should be made to minimize it.

    b.   **Intestinal illness**
Drinking water which is contaminated with soaps can cause diarrhea and other intestinal irritations.

  2. **Aesthetic impacts**
Who wants to drink water downstream of someone who has just washed in it with shampoo? Even if the physical impact is relatively small, who would enjoy the aesthetic or psychological impact? Wilderness is an area where human impact is relatively small; seeing soap suds floating down a stream does not fit this ideal.

  3. **Legal considerations**
In most areas, it is illegal to put any foreign substance into the water system.

B. **Bathing — How?**

  1. **Preparation**

    a.   Fill two or more billy cans (cook pots or other containers) with water.

    b.   Select a site at least 150 ft. (45 m.) from the water source with good drainage.

    c.   If possible, have a partner available to help.

  2. **Bathing**

    a.   Enter the lake or stream to get wet in preparation for bathing.

    b.   Walk up to the washing location and soap and wash thoroughly.

  3. **Rinsing**

    a.   Once thoroughly washed and ready to rinse, have a partner slowly pour water over head

and body, rinsing the soap off.
b.   If necessary, have a partner get more water to
     finish rinsing off.
c.   Once thoroughly rinsed with no trace of visible
     soap remaining, enter the stream or lake for a
     final rinse.

C.   **Washing Clothes — How?**
1.   **Preparation**
     Prepare as for a bath except a partner is not necessary.
2.   **Washing**
     a.   Rinse clothes thoroughly in a lake or stream but
          use no soap.
     b.   Take the clothes up to the washing site and wash
          them in a billy can, using soap as necessary.
3.   **Rinsing**
     a.   In a billy can of clean water, rinse the clothing.
          Keep replacing the soapy water with clean water
          until the clothing is completely rinsed. (It is not
          necessary to rinse clothing in a stream or lake.)
     b.   It is important to realize that most soaps do not
          rinse well in cold water and soap residue in
          clothing may cause skin irritation.
     c.   Hang clothing out to dry.
     d.   Use care in disposing of the soapy water –
          choose an area with good drainage at least 150
          ft. (45 m.) from your water source.

D.   **Bathing and Washing — When?**
1.   **Bathing**
     If possible, it is wise to bathe every day to help
     maintain spirits, sanitation, and good health. If
     bathing is not possible, try to wash the face daily
     and hands more frequently, especially before
     cooking.
2.   **Washing**
     Often, just rinsing clothes will help remove perspira-
     tion and body salts, although this does little to
     remove dirt and odor. Washing with soap can be
     done occasionally, but be sure to rinse thoroughly to
     prevent skin irritation due to soap residue.

IV. INSTRUCTIONAL STRATEGIES & MATERIALS:

A. **Timing**

This class is best demonstrated early in the trip to set a tone of bathing regularly and demonstrating care for the environment.

B. **Strategies**

1. Baths can be taken with swim suits on or males and females can go to different areas for privacy.
2. This may be a good time to discuss public nudity, as well as the course policy regarding coed bathing and the importance of being discrete with other groups and individuals.

C. **Materials**

1. Billy can (two or more)
2. Soap

2. Campsite Selection

I. **GOAL:** To have participants select, establish, maintain, and break down campsites with consideration for group safety, avoiding damage to equipment, and minimizing harm to the environment.

II. **OBJECTIVES:**
   A. Participants will be able to list the considerations in selecting a low-impact campsite.
   B. Participants will be able to list the considerations in selecting a safe and comfortable campsite.
   C. Participants will demonstrate an ability to establish a camp in relation to the group's physical and emotional state, time of day, and other factors.
   D. Participants will understand the role local rules and regulations play in determining campsite selection.
   E. Participants will be able to list the considerations in breaking camp.

III. **CONTENT:**
   A. **The Low-Impact Campsite**
       Selecting a low-impact campsite at first may appear to be determined by rules, but instead should be based on an ethic, using guidelines as a framework in making decisions. Low-impact campsite considerations include:
       1. **Established campsites vs. pristine campsites**
           One of the first decisions to be made is whether impact will be minimized by camping at an established campsite or at a pristine or "virgin" campsite where no one has ever camped before. WEA has no set policy regarding established vs. pristine campsites but offers these considerations:

© 1992
The Wilderness Education Association
P.O. Box 89
Saranac Lake, New York 12983
(518) 891-2915 ext. 254

a.   Selecting campsites which have never been used before provides a higher quality and more genuine wilderness experience.

    b.   Having participants select pristine campsites takes a higher level of decision making, thereby providing another opportunity to develop leadership skills.

    c.   Established campsites should perhaps be left for campers who may not have the knowledge or skills to select a pristine site.

    d.   Established campsites should be used when it is felt that using one will provide either a safer or more environmentally sound location.

2. **Aesthetics**

The group should camp out of sight and sound of trails, shorelines, and other groups because:

    a.   It provides a higher quality experience for others if they don't see evidence of another group camped there and increases the social/psychological carrying capacity of an area.

    b.   It is illegal to camp within these areas in most regions, unless the local agency has designated campsites within these limits.

3. **Water**

Can the group camp at the selected location and protect the quality of the water source?

4. **Ground cover**

    a.   Can the ground cover withstand the amount and type of use the group will give it?

    b.   Can tents be pitched and a campsite established without disturbing the existing cover (i.e., moving rocks, or logs, pulling up vegetation, etc.)? This is especially critical when canoe camping, since it is very easy to destroy vegetation along the shore when hauling canoes and packs out of the water.

    c.   Can the site that is chosen handle the amount of use expected?

    d.   Are participants watching where they walk to avoid trampling ferns, flowers, and other delicate flora? Encourage participants to "walk lightly."

5. **Wildlife**
   Will use of the site have an adverse effect on wildlife and their habits?
6. **Slope**
   Will the group subject the site to erosion?
7. **Wood**
   Can wood for fires be used without having an adverse impact on the area's fuel supply?

B. **Safety and Comfort**
   It is critical from a liability standpoint and for the group's emotional well-being, that the site is safe and reasonably comfortable. Safety and comfort considerations include:
   1. **Weather**
      Is the site reasonably protected from elements of wind, precipitation, lightning, and flash floods?
   2. **Water**
      Is a suitable water source within a reasonable distance?
   3. **Widowmakers** (a dead tree or tree limb(s) that could potentially fall and cause injury). Are tent sites free of dangerous widowmakers?
   4. **Slope**
      Can reasonably comfortable tentsites and meeting areas be found?
   5. **Aspect** (the direction the campsite faces). How is the camp's location in relation to the sun, weather, views, etc.?
   6. **Geology**
      Is the campsite safe from falling rocks, etc.?
   7. **Privacy**
      Is there sufficient space available to afford privacy for individuals in the group and the group as a whole (also considering social/psychological impact of those outside the group that may encounter the site).

C. **When to Camp**
   1. **Before the group is overtired**
      a. If the leader has to ask if the group is ready to camp, it is probably time to do so.
      b. Group members may be afraid to admit they are tired, or others may not realize how tired they are.

c.   The potential for accidents, injury, and environmental damage increases when the group is tired; therefore, if in doubt, set up camp.

2. **Before darkness**
      a.   Few enjoy setting up camp in the dark, especially after a hard day.
      b.   The potential for safety and environmental damage increases after sunset.
      c.   Setting up camp in the early afternoon allows the group to:
         • enjoy the area
         • explore
         • get personal and group chores done
         • replenish energy and enthusiasm
         • get a good campsite in crowded areas

D. **Rules and Regulations**
    1. Local rules and regulations are usually implemented to protect the wilderness user or the wilderness resource; therefore every attempt should be made to follow them.
    2. If rules are not followed by the group, a double standard results and sets a tone of "do as I say, not as I do."
    3. If for some reason rules are not followed, be sure to discuss the reason with the group so they understand the justification.
    4. *Discuss local rules and regulations pertaining to campsites at this time.*

E. **Breaking Camp**
    1. To make sure that every attempt has been made to minimize signs of the group's presence, when breaking camp it is the LOD's responsibility to check:
        • every tentsite
        • kitchen areas
        • meeting areas
        • the latrine
    2. Have campers restore trails and other areas to hide signs of the group's presence. Restoring should leave a natural look.

IV. INSTRUCTIONAL STRATEGIES & MATERIALS:

A. **Timing**

1. While safety and low-impact considerations in campsite selection need to be taught immediately, campsite selection as a class should be taught after students have had an opportunity to select campsites and have had a little experience with both good and bad campsites. This reinforces the information in this lesson and gives it more meaning.

2. Early safety and low-impact considerations can be taught informally on a small group basis, but it is essential to have a formal class on campsite considerations to reinforce this knowledge.

B. **Strategies**

1. In grizzly bear country or country where black bears present a problem:

   a. Avoid setting up tents in bear habitat or bedding areas. Bears are attracted to secure, cool areas that provide thick, low, ground cover (e.g., thick woods or brush, under deadfall, near water, etc.). Extreme care should be taken in choosing a site in bear country, since virtually all areas may be habitat (Peacock, 1990).

   b. Set up tent sites away from areas where food has been eaten, stored, or prepared. Also avoid putting tents between these areas and bear habitat.

   c. Where possible, group the tents together in a line so bears can easily avoid the area and not become inadvertently surrounded by tents.

C. **Activities**

1. Let the LOD or their delegate select the campsite and have the group critique it at the next debriefing.

2. Take the whole group through the campsite just before leaving and have them evaluate how well they camouflaged their sites and what could be done to improve it.

D. **Materials**

Campsite(s)

3. Clothing Selection

I. **GOAL**: To have participants select and properly use clothing appropriate for backcountry travel in temperate climate zones during the spring, summer, and fall seasons.

II. **OBJECTIVES**:
    A. Participants will understand and describe the major considerations that go into the selection of clothing for backcountry travel.
    B. Participants will understand and be able to discuss the positive and negative characteristics of the most common fabrics and materials used in backcountry clothing.
    C. Participants will understand and be able to explain the concepts of insulation, ventilation, and layering as they apply to the selection of clothing for backcountry travel.
    D. Participants will be able to make a list of clothing suitable for a backcountry expedition and justify each of their selections.

III. **CONTENT**:
    A. **Physiological Considerations**
        Backcountry travelers must select clothing which will allow them to maintain a stable body core temperature, dissipate excess body heat and moisture, and protect themselves from the elements.
        1. **Temperature control**
            Clothing must permit the body's core temperature to be maintained within a relatively narrow range above or below 98° for proper physical and mental functioning.

© 1992
The Wilderness Education Association
P.O. Box 89
Saranac Lake, New York 12983
(518) 891-2915 ext. 254

2. **Humidity control**
   Clothing must allow the water vapor produced by the body to dissipate readily from the body's surface.

3. **Protection from injury**
   Clothing should protect the wearer from common minor injuries associated with travel in the backcountry (e.g., sunburn, blisters, insect bites, skin irritation from poisonous plants, or briars, etc.).

B. **General Principles of Clothing Selection**
   1. **Clothing should be roomy and comfortable.**
      a. Clothing must allow for reasonable freedom of movement.
      b. Clothing must allow for unhindered blood circulation. Tightly bound elasticized cuffs around wrists or ankles should be avoided as they tend to restrict circulation.

   2. **Clothing must keep the wearer warm.**
      a. Some articles must be capable of providing the wearer with "insulation" (i.e., dead air space which creates a thermal barrier between the body of the wearer and the colder environment). The thermal conductance of the material should be low. Thermal conductance refers to the ability of the fabric to allow the transfer of heat. Thermal conductance is measured in kilocalories per square meter ($Kcal/m^2$). The larger the number, the better the conductor, and therefore the poorer its insulation ability.
      b. Clothing should be selected so that it can be "layered." Layering (i.e., the wearing of two or more lighter garments versus one heavy garment) allows the wearer to respond to changing environmental conditions and levels of exertion.
      c. Clothing must maintain its ability to insulate even when wet from perspiration or external sources of moisture.
      d. Clothing should have different adjustments to allow for ventilation (e.g., zippers, velcro, snaps, buttons).

   3. **Clothing should keep the wearer dry**
      a. Clothing should allow the wearer to "ventilate" excess body heat during periods of vigorous

activity. Garments should have easily accessible zippers, buttons, or velcro tabs which facilitate ventilation.

b. Inner layers of clothing should be of materials which absorb minimal amounts of moisture and which allow moisture to readily pass from the body's surface (e.g., wool, polypropylene, Thermax, Capilene).

c. Protective layers of outer clothing (i.e., rain or snow gear) should repel moisture to maintain the effectiveness of insulation (e.g., coated nylon, Gore-Tex).

d. All layers of clothing should dry rapidly.

e. Insulation layers should be knits or fabrics that "breathe" easily, allowing for the passage of body moisture.

4. **Clothing must be dependable**

a. Zippers, buttons, stitching, etc., should be of heavy duty quality that can withstand the rigors of wilderness travel.

b. External layers of clothing should be of reinforced fabric capable of withstanding heavy wear in areas such as elbows, knees, seat, etc.

5. **Clothing should be versatile and have multiple uses to minimize pack weight** (e.g., shorts doubling as swim suit, long john top as night shirt or insulation layer).

6. **Clothing should be lightweight and compressible.** One must be able to "stuff" clothes into sacks or in crevices within the pack.

7. **Clothing should be properly designed for its function** (e.g., external garments should have large pockets which are conveniently located and can be securely fastened).

8. **Clothing should be easy to maintain**

a. Inner garments should be relatively easy to launder and capable of withstanding repeated rinsings.

b. Clothing should not have extra decorations, zippers, or "doo-dads" which may rip, tear, or separate, compromising the usefulness of the garment.

C. **Clothing Materials and Their Characteristics**
1. **Wool**
Traditionally the most common insulating material found in the backcountry because of its distinct advantages over other natural fibers.
a. **Advantages of wool:**
(1) Wool is a poor thermal conductor (2 Kcal/ m²) thus a good insulator.
(2) Due to its unique structure, wool retains warmth when wet because closed air cells within the wool fiber provide insulation even when the outer surface of the fiber is soaked with water. In other words, wool provides effective insulation even when wet.
(3) Wool will dry via body heat while being worn.
(4) Wool clothing can be purchased relatively cheaply from second-hand stores or military surplus outlets.
(5) Tightly woven wool will shed snow and cut down on wind penetration.
(6) High quality wool containing lanolin absorbs relatively little moisture.
b. **Disadvantages of wool:**
(1) Coarse fibers may irritate sensitive skin.
(2) Wool will shrink if washed or dried in hot temperatures.
(3) It is difficult to completely dry heavier weaves.
(4) It is usually bulky and heavy and doesn't compress well.
2. **Cotton**
One of the most common and comfortable natural fibers in "civilian" clothing.
a. **Advantages of cotton:**
(1) It is very comfortable to the skin in warm weather because it is very breathable and conducts heat away from the body.
(2) It is readily available to purchase.
(3) It is easily laundered in all temperatures.
b. **Disadvantages of cotton:**
(1) It absorbs water readily (7% of its weight in moisture) from both the wearer and the

environment increasing conductive heat loss (Denner, 1990).

(2) It loses insulative value dramatically when wet because of its high level of moisture absorption.

(3) It is a good thermal conductor (6 Kcal/m^2) making it a poor insulator even when dry.

(4) It is very slow to dry.

(5) It tends to mildew under constant wet, humid conditions.

(6) It becomes heavy when wet.

(7) Cotton garments such as jeans, sweat pants, and sweat shirts are dangerous in the wilderness and should not be worn in chilly, wet, or windy weather. Cotton clothing that is damp or wet is a major contributor to hypothermia.

3. **Synthetic fibers**

a. **Modern polyester-based fibers fall into three general categories:**

(1) Insulating fabrics (e.g., polypropylene, pile, bunting, Thermax, Capilene, Polarlite, Polarplus, Synchilla, etc.)

(2) Insulating fills (e.g., Hollofill, Quallofill, Polarguard, Thinsulate, etc.)

(3) Shell fabrics (e.g., nylon taffeta, ripstop nylon, cordura, etc.)

b. **Uses of synthetic fabrics:**

(1) **Undergarments**: polypropylene and similar fibers are commonly used as inner layer undergarments and come in various weights for different activities.

(2) **Outergarments**: piles and bunting provide a middle insulating layer and are used for shirts, jackets, and pants. Insulating fills are used in outerwear layers in extreme cold or for sedentary activities.

(3) **External shell**: nylon and nylon blends provide windproof and waterproof garments depending on whether they are coated, uncoated, or bonded with some-

thing such as Gore-Tex to produce a specialty fabric.

(a) Uncoated nylon is usually tightly woven and resists wind penetration while still allowing body moisture to escape. Uncoated nylon may repel but will not stop penetration by rain or melting snow.

(b) Coated nylon is made essentially waterproof with a sealant such as urethane or neoprene. Moisture can neither pass in nor out of the garment. Such garments trap body moisture and will soak the wearer with perspiration if not well ventilated.

c. **Advantages of synthetic fabrics:**
   (1) They are very lightweight (a fraction of the weight of wool).
   (2) They absorb virtually no water (1% or less).
   (3) They are poor thermal conductors (1.5 Kcal/m²) and thus conserve heat.
   (4) They dry very rapidly while being worn.
   (5) They feel comfortable against the skin of most people.
   (6) They are non-allergenic.
   (7) They are less prone to mildew and rot than natural fibers.
   (8) They come in a variety of weights, blends, colors, and styles.

d. **Disadvantages of synthetic fabrics:**
   (1) They are relatively expensive.
   (2) Synthetic fibers will melt or burn readily when exposed to sparks or flame.
   (3) Synthetic insulators without nylon shells offer minimal protection from the wind.
   (4) With a few exceptions, synthetic fibers tend to retain body odors even after laundering.
   (5) Some synthetic insulators do not withstand abrasion well and must be reinforced by nylon shells.

(6)   Some synthetics are sensitive to extreme heat, so caution must be used in laundering.

4. **Fabric blends**

Fabric blends are a combination of nylon, cotton, wool, polypropylene, and other fibers.

  a. **Advantages of fabric blends:** When properly constructed, such garments combine the best qualities of each fabric, frequently adding to the strength and abrasion resistance of the garment.

  b. **Disadvantages of fabric blends:** Blending often results in garments which combine the weaknesses of each fabric. Blends containing cotton absorb water readily and freeze in cold weather.

5. **Breathable waterproof fabrics**

These are fabrics coated or bonded with a micro-porous membrane which keeps the larger droplets of rain out but lets the smaller water vapors escape.

  a. **Advantages of breathable waterproof fabrics:**

    (1)   They allow body moisture to escape while preventing external moisture from penetrating the garment.

    (2)   They stop wind penetration very well.

  b. **Disadvantages of breathable waterproof fabrics:**

    (1)   Good quality garments are very expensive.

    (2)   There is little consensus on the effectiveness of these garments (i.e., some feel they do not breathe sufficiently during heavy exertion or not at all in the rain).

    (3)   Soiling of garment reduces breathability.

    (4)   Special care must be taken in laundering.

    (5)   Many brand names provide "lifetime" warranties. Unfortunately, these are of little use when they fail in the field.

    (6)   After repeated use, the finish needs to be re-coated with a scotch-guard product to maintain waterproofing.

D. **Clothing List for Backcountry Travel** (suitable for 3-season camping)

1. *Boxer shorts* (2 pair): lightweight, easy to launder, prevent chafing between legs.

2. *Synthetic or synthetic/wool blend long underwear top* (1 or 2): serves as pajama top or cool weather inner insulation layer.

3. *Long sleeve, cotton/polyester, light weave dress shirt*: warm-weather garment, dries fast, protects against insects, should have breast pockets that button.

4. *Long underwear bottom* (optional for people who sleep or hike cold): synthetic or synthetic/wool blend.

5. *Wool or pile trousers* (1 pair): 100% wool, synthetic/wool blend, or synthetic pile. Fit should permit freedom of movement and be large enough to allow middle or outer layers to be tucked in.

6. *Shorts* (1 or 2 pair): nylon or nylon blend with a loose fit for comfort while walking. Nylon shorts dry readily and can double as swim trunks and underwear.

7. *Heavy C.P.O. type wool or pile shirt* (1): should be long in torso, have a synthetic neck or wrist lining, and button breast pockets.

8. *Sweaters* (2): wool, pile, or bunting.

9. *Rainwear* (1): coated nylon or Gore-Tex. Ideally, it should extend below the crotch and have ample ventilation. Hooded parkas, although standard in most rainwear, are a matter of personal preference since hoods can restrict visibility and hearing.

10. *Nylon wind parka/shirt* (1): should be lightweight and roomy enough to wear sweaters underneath. Pockets are convenient. Good for warm "buggy" weather. Gore-Tex parka may be adequate for both wind and rain.

11. *Nylon wind pants* (1 pair): protect legs from wind and insects. Can be layered over wool pants or worn over undershorts in warm weather. Pockets are very useful, while a drawstring closure at the waist makes for easy adjustment. Zippered legs are helpful for putting on over boots.

12. *Wool, synthetic, or wool/blend cap* (1): insulates head; should cover ears and back of neck.

13. *Wool, synthetic, or wool/blend gloves* (1 pair).

14. *Wool, synthetic, or wool/blend mittens* (1 pair): layer over gloves in cold weather.
15. *Cotton work gloves* (1 pair): use around fire to protect hands from drying heat; also use as pot holders.
16. *Wide brim felt hat* (1): wide brim keeps rain and sun out of eyes and off neck.
17. *Baseball cap* (optional): keeps sun out of eyes and provides style and comfort.
18. *Bandanas* (2 or more): several extra large cotton/polyester handkerchiefs; multitude of uses.
19. *Belt or suspenders*
20. *Sunglasses* (1 pair): essential for protection from sun and glare off sand, water, or ice.
21. *Footwear*
    a. **Socks** (4-6 pair): should be medium to heavy wool/synthetic blend socks. Two pair of socks should normally be worn with boots to minimize blisters. While two pair of socks of equal weight are more versatile (i.e., inner and outer socks can be readily exchanged) a light synthetic inner sock has gained in popularity due to its ability to prevent blisters and wick moisture away from the foot.
    b. **Sneakers**: lightweight, nylon sneakers, canvas wading shoes, or other lightweight footwear is a must for around camp. They should fit over heavy socks.
    c. **Boots — General Guidelines:**
       (1) Weight of the boot should be appropriate for the ruggedness of the terrain and for the size and weight of the packer. Easy trails and light packs call for lighter weight boots. Big packs and rough trails require boots of sturdier construction.
       (2) Boots must support the ankle and protect the sole of the foot. Stiff, full leather heavy boots maximize ankle support for heavy loads over rocky, rugged terrain. Lightweight, flexible Gore-Tex-lined boots are appropriate for shorter trips, light packs, and relatively easy trails.
       (3) Boots must fit the packer's foot comfortably when wearing two pairs of hiking

socks and allow for foot expansion late in the day under heavy loads. Two pair of socks minimize blisters and maximize wicking action of moisture away from the foot.

(4) Boots must be well constructed. Check to see that stitching, grommets, seams, sole, and insoles are of good quality material capable of withstanding harsh treatment.

(5) Boots should "breathe." Waterproof rubber boots are a poor choice for three-season hiking.

d. **Fitting boots**

(1) Put the boot on with the foot bare or with a liner sock only.

    (a) Slide the foot forward in the boot.

    (b) Should be able to insert two fingers between the back of the boot and the achilles tendon (the back of the foot).

(2) Put on two pair of socks of the type to be used.

    (a) The sides of the foot should just touch the inner sides of the boot.

    (b) Toes should be able to wiggle comfortably.

    (c) One finger should fit between the heel of the foot and the back of the boot.

(3) Lace the boot comfortably and walk.

    (a) The heel should lift just slightly off the bottom of the boot.

    (b) The arch of the inner sole should conform to the arch of the foot.

    (c) The ball of the foot must conform to the slight depression in the inner sole.

(4) Kick the boot toe against a solid object several times. The big toe should not come in contact with the front of the boot.

(5) If the feet are of uneven size, always fit the longer foot. Use an extra thick insole or extra sock for the smaller foot.

IV. **INSTRUCTIONAL STRATEGIES & MATERIALS:**
   A. **Timing**
       1. Clothing acquisition is usually reviewed either through written communication or in a pre-trip orientation. It is essential for staff to ensure that participants are properly outfitted. This is most often done through a pre-trip clothing and equipment check.
       2. Information concerning clothing selection is reinforced informally throughout the course. A more formal presentation on the subject may be part of a classroom course or held near the end of the WEA course when participants have had the opportunity to formulate their own views on their personal clothing selection and compare them to others.

   B. **Strategies**
       1. This lesson may be taught early on a course as an instructor-directed lecture/demonstration in which each article of clothing is presented and the rationale for its selection explained.
       2. Later in the course, a participant-oriented lesson may prove more fruitful in reinforcing the reasons for clothing selection. Some ideas for generating participant discussion might include:
           a. Participants present an article of gear to the group and present reasons for its selection.
           b. Create a small group skit involving "uninformed" campers packing for a trip. Ask audience to comment on their obvious blunders.
           c. Write and read a short story describing backpackers on the trail who get into trouble (hypothermia, blisters, ankle sprains, etc.) because of poor clothing choice. Have participants write down "what they did wrong" and use this as a basis for discussion.

C. **Materials**
1. Boxer shorts
2. Long underwear top
3. Long sleeve cotton/polyester, light weave, dress shirt
4. Long underwear bottom
5. Trousers
6. Shorts
7. Heavy C.P.O. type wool or pile shirt
8. Sweater
9. Rainwear
10. Wind parka/shirt
11. Wind pants
12. Wool cap
13. Liner gloves
14. Mittens
15. Cotton work gloves
16. Wide brim felt hat
17. Baseball cap
18. Bandana
19. Belt or suspender
20. Sunglasses
21. Footwear: socks, sneakers, boots

4. Decision Making

I. **GOAL:** To provide participants with a background of decision-making theory and introduce them to its field application.

II. **OBJECTIVES:**
   A. Participants will be able to define the decision-making process.
   B. Participants will be able to list and describe the steps in the decision-making process.
   C. Participants will be able to distinguish between "simple" and "complex" decision-making situations and describe the characteristics of each.
   D. Participants will be able to discuss the role which decision-making activities play in WEA's leadership training.
   E. Participants will be able to demonstrate the application of the decision-making process in simulated exercises.
   F. Participants will be able to discuss the interdisciplinary nature of the decision-making process and its application in non-wilderness settings.

III. **CONTENT:**
   A. **Variability in Decision Making**
      1. **All decision-making situations are not created equal**
         a. Every decision-making situation comes with its own set of circumstances and variables which make it unique. No matter how often a decision-making situation may arise, some variable has changed since the last time it was encountered. If nothing else, the variable of time has changed. It is important that decision makers recognize this variability and take it into account when making or evaluating decisions.
         b. Decision-making situations range in complexity. Some decisions are very simple and easily

made. Other decisions are exceedingly complex and difficult. Every decision lies somewhere along an imaginary continuum that ranges from simple to complex. Knowing the characteristics of simple and complex decisions can be helpful in developing strategies for responding effectively to different decision-making situations. It also may have implications for the style of decision making employed in each situation.

2. **Simple decisions**
   a. **Characteristics of simple decision-making situations:**
      (1) The challenge confronting the decision makers is clearly understood by all and everyone involved understands what they are trying to accomplish.
      (2) The information required to make the decision is available, unambiguous, and the outcomes are predictable within a reasonable range of probability.
      (3) The range of possible choices or options is fairly obvious and within the common experience of those affected by the decision.
      (4) The time frame within which the decision is made is not unduly pressing. Participants feel they have time to give each option appropriate consideration.
      (5) The skills needed to make the decision are primarily analytic. Decision makers can objectively balance the positive and negative implications of each course of action.
      (6) The decision and its outcomes do not challenge or threaten the core values or interests of the participants. Simple decisions are not commonly perceived as life-changing, nor do they force people to reexamine who or what they are, or what they stand for.
      (7) The maturity and/or level of experience of the group is appropriate to deal with the potential outcomes of the decisions and the processes needed to implement them.

b. **Observations on making simple decisions:**
(1) Simple decisions rarely take much time and often take little effort.
(2) Since group members do not usually see simple decisions as very threatening, their personal investment in the process need not be very high. Frequently, group members are very content to turn simple decision making over to others (e.g., a committee or a leader).
(3) Reducing the number of participants in the process of simple decision making conserves valuable time and the emotional resources of the group. Imagine the frustration of a daily full-group debate over when to have lunch!
(4) Experience in simple decision making can lead to a pattern of decision-maker response which proves useful as similar challenges arise. In effect, a procedure for handling specific types of decisions may emerge, which greatly facilitates the process.
(5) While procedures are useful, the group must beware of relying on them too much. Procedures have a way of hardening into bureaucratic dogma that soon impedes quality decision making. Take heed!

3. **Complex decisions**
a. **Characteristics of complex decision-making situations**
(1) Uncertainty is the common denominator which distinguishes complex from simple decision making. To the extent that uncertainty affects any level of the process (information, options, or outcomes), simple decisions become more difficult and success less predictable.
(2) Given the fluid nature of outdoor adventure activities, many if not most decisions encountered by outdoor leaders are complex.

b. **Observations on complex decisions:**
   (1) As decisions become more complex and the implications of their outcomes more uncertain, group members are more likely to want to have some control over the process. While accommodating this impulse may not always be possible (as in a life-threatening emergency), decision makers are well advised to be aware of its existence and proceed accordingly.
   (2) Brainstorming is one technique which decision makers may use to reduce uncertainty when facing complex decision-making situations. (See section C. 3. later in this chapter.)
c. **The role of judgment in complex decision-making:**
   (1) When information is incomplete and knowledge uncertain, analysis must give way to judgment as the driving force of decision making. Complex decisions rarely yield to "correct" answers or solutions. Instead, options are evaluated in terms of probability rather than certainty of success.
   (2) Judgment is the accumulated wisdom we glean from past experience and apply to present problems. Decision makers with good judgment are able to increase the probability of successful problem solving because they understand how to process their experience and apply it to the unique circumstances of each new challenge. Judgment gives one a perspective — a lens through which events are viewed in sharper focus and with greater clarity.
   (3) Judgment is required at all stages of the decision-making process.
   (4) Judgment requires processing experience and adopting new behaviors as a result of that experience.
   (5) "The feature of the WEA curriculum that distinguishes it the most from all other

outdoor leadership development programs is its emphasis upon theoretical and
experience-based judgment, and on
decision-making ability as the necessary
foundation of all outdoor leadership
competence. As the core is to the apple, so
is judgment and decision-making ability to
outdoor leadership" (Cockrell, 1991, p. 13).

B. **Defining the decision-making process**
1. **The decision-making process is a series of steps**
    towards making a rational choice among options,
    for the purpose of realizing an objective. The
    process, as outlined below, is appropriate for almost
    any decision-making situation regardless of its
    complexity. The manner in which decision makers
    choose to engage the process will obviously depend
    upon the situation.
2. **Characteristics of the process**
    a. The process of decision making is the product
        of rational thought as opposed to the exercise of
        preference. The logical steps taken to reach a
        decision should be easily understood to an
        independent observer.
        (1) For example, the choice of the evening's
            meal is an exercise of preference and does
            not necessarily have a basis in logic (and is
            an example of a simple decision). The
            selection of a route to a given campsite
            should be a product of rational thought,
            the logic of which should include the
            consideration of time, terrain, physical
            condition of the group, and other factors.
            (This serves as an example of a more
            complex decision.)
        (2) It should be noted that the emphasis on
            rational thought in this process does not
            discount the role individual experience
            plays, nor preclude the use of hunches and
            "feelings" which may be based upon that
            experience.
    b. The need for a decision comes from a recogni-
        tion that a difference exists between that which

is and that which is not desirable. The desire to meet some objective is always implied. Without some recognized objective, no decision is necessary or possible.

c.   Decision making always involves a choice and implies the consideration of more than one option. If only one course of action exists in a given situation, then no decision is required.

d.   Decision making implies action. The process of decision making is incomplete without an attempt to implement the decision.

e.   Decision making always takes place within a specific historical, physical, and cultural "context." This context consists of the physical, cultural, and philosophical elements which contribute to the setting in which the decision is made. Such contributing elements include the temperature, altitude, and topography of the area; the age, gender mix, and ethnicity of the group; or the objectives of the individuals, group, or agency which is included in the expedition.

f.   The use of the decision-making process does not guarantee the outcome of a specific action. However, consistent application of the process, tempered by the judgment that comes from experience, significantly increases the odds of meeting objectives.

C.   **Steps in the decision-making process**
1.   **Framing the problem — the challenge**
    a.   **Recognition** – Decision making starts when the group perceives a difference between what is and what is not desirable.
    b.   **Motivation** – The group must desire to seek out and choose a course of action which will change the situation.
    c.   **Goal setting** – The group must identify its objectives or goals so that everyone will be working toward a common end.

In the "Decision at High Mountain" scenario (which can be found in the appendix at the end of this chapter), the process begins when the group recognizes that it has inadvertently gotten lost and is not proceeding along a trail that will take them home. Clearly the group is motivated to improve their situation. The group agrees that they wish to get home as soon as possible without unnecessary risk to their survival.

2. **Analysis of relevant concerns**
   A systematic consideration of all the factors which may bear on the situation.
   a. **Gathering of facts:** The collection of information that can be confirmed by an independent observer. These "facts" are viewed by the decision makers as empirically true. In the "Decision at High Mountain" scenario, some of the "facts" are:
      (1) There are two trail routes out to their car.
      (2) Their clothing includes blue jeans, cotton hooded sweat shirts, wool clothing and "Mickey Mouse" boots.
      (3) Their equipment includes a mountain tent, sleeping bags, backpacking stove, one map, and one compass.
      (4) They have to be back to work on Monday.
      (5) They have left vague emergency information.
   b. **Reviewing assumptions:** An examination of information and/or beliefs which decision makers accept as true but which cannot be proven or verified. In the "Decision at High Mountain" scenario, some of the assumptions might be:
      (1) The weather will remain seasonably unpredictable.
      (2) It will be a while before anyone starts looking for them.
      (3) Their parents will worry if they don't come home on time.
      (4) They may be disciplined at work for absence.
   c. **Recognizing constraints:** A recognition of the limitations which the present circumstances impose. In the "Decision at High Mountain" scenario, some of the constraints which might be recognized are:
      (1) Availability of food
      (2) Weather conditions

(3) Time

(4) Experience and expertise of group members

d. **Understanding values:** An attempt to understand the influence of those ideas, beliefs, and goals that are considered by the group to be most important to the group's success or survival. In the "Decision at High Mountain" scenario, some of the values of the group might be:

(1) Sense of responsibility to employer

(2) Consideration of family feeling and emotions

(3) Loyalty to all the members of the party

(4) Commitment to the survival of all party members

e. **Recognizing group dynamics:** An effort to predict the impact which potential courses of action may have on individual morale and the ability of the group to function effectively as a unit. In the "Decision at High Mountain" scenario, some factors involving group dynamics might include:

(1) The least experienced group member did not follow the advice of the more experienced group members.

(2) The individual who is least prepared is also the youngest.

(3) There was tension within the group on the ride to the trailhead because of the factors cited above.

3. **Identifying options and brainstorming**

Brainstorming is a group problem-solving technique in which group members are encouraged to spontaneously contribute any idea that comes into their heads.

a. **Advantages of brainstorming**

(1) It broadens the base of experience from which to draw constructive ideas.

(2) It improves the probability that all options will be thoroughly considered.

(3) It encourages a sense of participant "ownership" of the final decision.

b. **Considerations when brainstorming**

(1) Brainstorming is a skill which takes time and practice to develop.

(2)   Brainstorming requires a high degree of tolerance from all participants. To be effective, a brainstorming session must be governed by the attitude that "anything is possible." All ideas must be afforded equal acceptance.

      (3)   Brainstorming usually requires at least one person to play the role of facilitator encouraging the sharing of ideas, and restraining the impulse to criticize or discount.

      (4)   Brainstorming may lead to an outcome which is the product of "group think" in which the power of peer pressure inadvertently squelches independent thought or dissent. The facilitator must be vigilant in this regard and sometimes act as a "devil's advocate."

4.   **Formulating and weighing options**
The examination of the positive and negative consequences of potential courses of action. In the "Decision at High Mountain" scenario, some of the options and their advantages and disadvantages might be:

a.   Return to and spend the night at Lake Clear lean-to.
   (1)   Advantage: minimal travel after dark.
   (2)   Disadvantage: will not return to work on time.

b.   Walk out to trail head via High Pass Trail.
   (1)   Advantages: they might get home that night.
   (2)   Disadvantages: they might get lost due to unfamiliarity with the trail.

c.   Remain in place and set up camp.
   (1)   Advantages: minimizes risk of hypothermia or exhaustion.
   (2)   Disadvantages: will not get home on time and family will worry.

d.   Walk out to trailhead via Lake Clear Trail.
   (1)   Advantages: familiar terrain.
   (2)   Disadvantages: longest route to travel.

5.   **Contingency plan**
At this point in the decision-making process, it is appropriate to identify a contingency plan by

outlining the "what if's" (alternatives) of each option. As an example, suppose a group is deciding whether or not to take a trailless hike to a marked trail which will lead to their campsite. Included in their decision-making process should be a plan (alternative) to answer the question, "What if we don't find the marked trail by dark?"

6. **Making the decision**

   a. Decision makers will use the decision-making process differently, depending on the unique circumstances of each situation. In general, these methods break down into four broad categories which closely parallel leadership styles discussed in the "Leadership" lesson.

   b. The autocratic method. One or a few individuals make the decision for the remainder of the group.

   c. The democratic method. Group members are encouraged to offer input. A tally of opinion (e.g., voting, majority rule) is implied.

   d. The laissez-faire method. Decision making by each individual in the group.

   e. The consensus method. All group members discuss options until unanimity is achieved.

7. **Implementing the decision**

   a. Once a decision is made, its successful implementation is usually an issue of effective management practices and procedures.

   b. Considerations for effective implementation include:

      (1) Communication – Everyone must understand at all times what they are to do and why they are to do it.

      (2) Delegation – Everyone involved should have specific tasks for which they are personally responsible.

      (3) Accountability – Everyone recognizes the value of their contribution to the success of the whole.

8. **Evaluation**

   This is the process by which participants determine what has been learned from the decision-making experience. By incorporating these understandings in future decisions, participants develop judgment. This step in the process is critical to the development of judgment in the WEA curriculum; the decision-making process is not complete until it is evaluated. The theme that runs throughout the entire curriculum process is the explanation of why an action should be, is, or was taken, why it was performed in the way it was, and in what way the action might be improved now or for similar situations in the future (Cockrell, 1991).

This is an appropriate time to discuss and evaluate the group's responses to the "Decision at High Mountain" scenario.

D. **Decision Making as Part of WEA Leadership Training**
   1. **Decision-making theory presentation**
      This presentation lays the foundation for understanding the concepts used in decision making.
   2. **Journals**
      Writing journals encourages participants to formally identify and analyze decisions made during the course.
   3. **Debriefings**
      Daily group debriefings give participants the opportunity to share and reflect on their analysis of decisions that have been made.
   4. **Instructor observation**
      Instructor observations provide participants with feedback concerning their progress in mastering the decision-making process.
   5. **Peer evaluation**
      Peer evaluation affords participants additional feedback from the group concerning their decision-making performance.

E. **The Interdisciplinary Nature of Decision Making**
   1. Participants should understand that the decision-making process itself is a system of thought which can be applied in any situation, regardless of circumstance.
   2. Participants should recognize that the processes of decision making developed in this course have application outside of a wilderness setting. The decision-making process can readily be applied in

non-wilderness situations, such as school, home, business, etc.

3. Experiences on the course should be interpreted metaphorically. The "metaphoric experience" is defined as an experience in one situation which has meaning and application in many other situations. The accumulation of many "metaphoric experiences," coupled with an ability to apply them successfully in new situations, is generally recognized as a defining characteristic of leaders possessing good judgment.

4. The leadership experiences encountered on a WEA course will train participants in a pattern of behavior which is useful in other wilderness situations. The responsibilities of a leader on a four-day expedition are essentially the same as those on a 35-day expedition.

IV. **INSTRUCTIONAL STRATEGIES & MATERIALS:**
A. **Timing**
This class should be taught no later than early in the second week of the course. (Wilderness Education Association courses are four to five weeks long.) If possible, it should be taught in the classroom before the start of the course and applied immediately once the course begins.

B. **Strategies**
1. **Theory** – The theory component is usually taught in a formal, outdoor classroom setting.
   a. Lecture
   b. Simulation
      (1) The "Decision at High Mountain" simulation (included in the appendix at the end of this chapter) can be used as a basis for discussion of the steps of the decision-making process. It is strongly suggested that participants have a thorough understanding of the scenario before the class begins.
      (2) Instructors may choose to use real-life situations in the field as a basis for discussion. Instructors should prepare their own analyses before class so that classes focus on the process, not the problem.

2. **Application** – The process should be applied through the everyday activities encountered in the course. Instructors can facilitate this through reinforcement and proper use of the evaluation process. The application occurs primarily through the following:
   a. Teachable moments
   b. Leader of the Day (LOD) experiences
3. **Evaluation** – Proper evaluation of the process is critical to insure that participants can understand and apply it. Evaluation is included in:
   a. Debriefings
   b. Journals
   c. Instructor evaluation
   d. Peer evaluation

"Decision At High Mountain"

Early on the morning of November 29th, Bob, Sue, and Mark headed into the High Mountain Wilderness Area on their third backpacking trip together. The weather was crisp and cool, with daytime highs in the 30s and the thermometer dipping into the teens at night. There were two inches of snow on the ground with a possibility of additional accumulation over the weekend.

Bob, 21 and Sue, 22 were well dressed for the outing in wool pants and shirts, and rubberized, insulated, winter hiking boots. Both were well equipped with good quality synthetic insulated sleeping bags and insulated sleeping pads. Mark,18 however, was not so well prepared. Although none of the hikers were highly experienced, Mark had only been backpacking on two previous occasions and was not yet ready to spend the money necessary for the proper gear. Sitting in Bob's suburban New Jersey home, Sue and Bob had pleaded with Mark to outfit himself properly. Nonetheless, when they met early Saturday morning, Mark appeared decked in blue jeans, cotton thermal longjohns, a hooded cotton sweatshirt, cotton tube socks, and leather workboots. He carried his gear in a borrowed, ill-fitted backpack and intended to sleep in a goosedown sleeping bag on an air mattress. The group would sleep together in Sue's three-person mountain tent.

Although the three had to be back at work early Monday, it was the last thing on their mind as they sped along the interstate highway on their six hour drive. Bob casually shared with Sue that he forgot to tell his parents exactly where he was going and Sue admitted she hadn't told her parents either. Mark spoke up saying, "Don't worry I told my parents we were going backpacking in the Adirondacks and not to worry, we'd be back by 11:00 p.m." The discussion turned to Mark's reluctance to acquire the proper clothing and equipment, creating a level of tension in the group which would last the weekend. The discussion ended as Bob pulled into the "Complete Backpacker" store to buy some new batteries for his flashlight before heading to the nearby trailhead.

© 1992
The Wilderness Education Association
P.O. Box 89
Saranac Lake, New York 12983
(518) 891-2915 ext. 254

The three hiked up the Lake Clear trail that Saturday afternoon with the intention of staying overnight at the lake and returning to their car the next day. Although the trail to the lake was over four miles long, the terrain was relatively easy and the three friends reached their destination by early afternoon. After setting up camp and eating dinner, the three settled into their tent for a well-deserved rest. As the night sky darkened and the thermometer dipped, a gentle snow began to fall.

Bob was the first to awaken on Sunday morning to a trackless, white world covered by the accumulation of the previous evening's flurries. Finally emerging from their respective cocoons at about 8:30 a.m., the campers set to the task of preparing a hot breakfast. After a breakfast of oatmeal and hot chocolate, the three stayed in their sleeping bags enjoying the warmth and friendly conversation. Around noon, they decided to have a hot lunch before heading back to their car. Much to their dismay, they found their otherwise dependable back-packing stove extremely difficult to light. Indeed, even after a frustrating hour of tinkering, the stove would only produce a very weak, short-lived flame. Finally, despairing of any progress, they gave up on the stove and munched on available pre-packaged granola bars and gulped down some nearly frozen water.

By 1:30 p.m., all three were packed and ready to head back on the trail home. Talking excitedly about the beauty of the new fallen snow and without paying any great heed to the few trail markers on the trees, the party moved out in what they thought was the direction from which they had come. After 30 minutes on the trail, Bob remarked how different everything looked from the day before. Sue mentioned that they should be more attentive to the trail markers since they no longer had the footprints of earlier hikers to follow as they had the previous day. Mark said that he couldn't remember the last time he had seen a trail marker. Within another 15 minutes, it became obvious to all that they were not exactly sure of their location.

Since Bob had the only map and compass in the group, he tried to figure out where they were. Though he had some elementary training in orienteering, it soon was obvious that his skills were not equal to the task at hand. Figuring that the trail had to be close by, they decided to spread out and look for markers. Within a few minutes, they discovered a marker of the appropriate color and headed down the trail with renewed confidence.

The three continued to hike for another 45 minutes when Bob remarked that he could see a trail sign in the distance. Hustling over to the sign, they read to their great chagrin:

"Trailhead via High Pass Trail 3.6 miles"

"Trailhead via Lake Clear Trail 7 miles"

"Lake Clear Lean-to 2.9 miles"

Their hearts sank as they realized they had been walking in the wrong direction all morning. Now, at 3:30 p.m. on Sunday afternoon with darkness only an hour away, they faced a decision. High Pass Trail was a direct route to the car but a quick glance at the map revealed it involved a 500-foot gain in elevation. Returning to the trailhead by the route they had just traveled would take them past Lake Clear lean-to on a familiar trail, but would mean nearly 3½ more miles of trail.

What should they do?

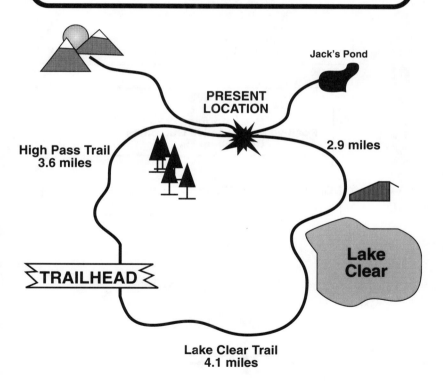

DECISION AT HIGH MOUNTAIN MAP

Jack's Pond

PRESENT
LOCATION

2.9 miles

High Pass Trail
3.6 miles

Lake
Clear

TRAILHEAD

Lake Clear Trail
4.1 miles

The Decision-Making Process

CONTEXT

IDENTIFY the PROBLEM

CLARIFICATION and ANALYSIS

Gather Facts
Examine Assumptions
Recognize Constraints
Understand Values
Consider Group Dynamics

C O N T E X T

OPTIONS

Brainstorming
Positive and Negative Outcomes
Contingencies

C O N T E X T

| OPTION 1 | OPTION 2 | OPTION 3 |

DECISION

IMPLEMENTATION

EVALUATION

CONTEXT

5. Environmental Ethics and Backcountry Conservation Practices

The authors would like to recognize the contributions of Dr. David Cockrell and his chapter on "Environmental Ethics and Backcountry Conservation Practices" which can be found in "The Wilderness Educator: The Wilderness Education Association Curriculum Guide."

I.   **GOAL**: To have participants develop and apply an appropriate standard of backcountry environmental ethics.

II. **OBJECTIVES**:

A.   Participants will be able to describe backcountry conservation practices as they relate to travel, campsite selection and use, stoves and cooking, and sanitation.

B.   Participants will be able to discuss the consequences of individual and group behavior on the quality of the outdoor experience.

C.   Participants will be able to discuss the concept of ethics as it relates to the natural environment and wilderness travel.

D.   Participants will be able to discuss their personal philosophy as it relates to backcountry conservation practices.

E.   Participants will be able to describe the implications their personal environmental philosophy has for their actions as citizens of the world.

III. **CONTENT**:

Since much of this content will be generated from participants reflecting on their experiences during the course, the range of potential topics for discussion is endless. The following outline is therefore presented in a question/answer format which is meant to generate discussion. See the diagram entitled "Environmental Ethics: A Progression" at the end of this chapter for a schematic representation of this approach.

© 1992
The Wilderness Education Association
P.O. Box 89
Saranac Lake, New York 12983
(518) 891-2915 ext. 254

A. **Observation/Recognition**
1. What kinds of backcountry conservation behavior have we observed while on this course? *Participants should be encouraged to note the full range of behavior they have seen.*
2. *Discussion leaders might use the following questions to guide discussion through various categories of backcountry behavior.*
    a. What evidence have we seen of human behavior while walking on the trail?
        (1) Litter
        (2) Tree blazing
        (3) Shortcutting of trails across switchbacks
        (4) Trail erosion
        (5) The absence of these signs
    b. What evidence have we seen of behavior in selecting campsites?
        (1) Concentrated destruction of plants and soil surface
        (2) Sites located immediately adjacent to water
        (3) Sites on the trail or in the middle of scenic areas
        (4) The absence of these signs
    c. What evidence have we seen of behavior regarding the use of fire?
        (1) Indiscriminate tree cutting
        (2) Scorched rocks
        (3) Multiple fire sites
        (4) Discarded fuel canisters
        (5) The absence of these signs
    d. What evidence have we seen of behavior regarding personal and group sanitation and hygiene?
        (1) Toilet paper and human waste
        (2) Soap scum in water
        (3) Food waste on the ground or in the water
        (4) The absence of these

B. **Application/Analysis**
1. Is there any pattern to the evidence of environmental behavior that we have seen on this trip?

a.   Yes. Clearly some people have chosen to behave in a way which leaves obvious evidence of their presence in the backcountry.

      b.   No. Although we can't see the impact of their passing, it is prudent to assume that many people traveled through this area leaving very little evidence behind.

2.   Are the behaviors we have seen strictly the result of individual action?

      a.   Yes. Someone either did or did not choose to act in a way which minimized their impact on the environment. Each individual contributes in their own way to the conditions we see in the backcountry.

      b.   No. People often travel in groups and the collective attitude/behavior of the group is more than the sum of the attitudes/behaviors of its members. People will do things as a member of a group that they would never think of doing as an individual.

3.   What are the consequences of these patterns of behavior (i.e., minimizing vs. ignoring one's impact on the environment)?

      a.   Behaviors which minimize impact on the environment may result in:

          (1)   Preservation of the "natural" character of an area for an extended period of time.

          (2)   Preservation of the quality/purity of the natural resources of an area for an extended period of time.

          (3)   Increase in the capacity of an area to support recreational use for an extended period of time.

      b.   Behaviors which ignore impact on the environment of an area may result in:

          (1)   Rapid deterioration of the "natural" character of an area over a short period of time.

          (2)   Rapid deterioration of the quality/purity of the natural resources of the area over a short period of time.

          (3)   Decrease in the capacity of an area to support recreational use in a short period of time.

4. Why do people adopt such patterns of behavior?
   a. Degree of education
   b. Appreciation of, and concern for the "natural" environment
   c. Desire for comfort or convenience
   d. Sensitivity to the impact of actions on others
   e. History of exposure to the out-of-doors
   f. Family background
5. What is the significance of these patterns?
   a. What can we recognize about those people who do not practice minimum impact camping techniques?
      (1) Some do not know about these techniques.
      (2) Some do know of these techniques but will not use them because they are not convinced of their necessity.
      (3) Some do know of these techniques but do not use them consistently for a variety of reasons. Many of these people do not consciously consider the consequences of their actions or do not believe that their individual behavior is significant.
   b. Do the actions of these people tell us anything about their values?
      Yes. Their behavior reveals their values (i.e., the ideas, beliefs, or types of behavior which they consider to be most important in guiding their life decisions). These actions tell us that they do not value the wilderness or the wilderness experience as much as those who do practice minimum impact techniques.
   c. What can we know about those people who do practice minimum impact camping techniques?
      (1) Since the practice of minimum impact techniques requires a conscious effort, it is safe to assume that these people have chosen to use these techniques for specific reasons.
      (2) It is evident that people using minimum impact techniques are aware of the consequences of their actions on the wilderness and the wilderness experience. Since their behavior is specifically in-

tended to preserve wilderness and enhance the wilderness experience, it is safe to assume that they value both highly. It is their concern for wilderness that has caused them to consciously restrict their own freedom of action in the backcountry for the sake of preserving it for themselves and others.

C. **Synthesis – A Land Ethic**
  1. **Definition of ethics:** A code of voluntary restrictions of individual freedom agreed upon by members of a society for the good of the community; conforming to the standards of conduct of a given profession.
     a. Ethics are socially derived (i.e., learned from the surrounding culture. For instance, parents teach their children to be responsible, cooperative, and obedient in order to help maintain harmony within the family. Certain actions are considered "right" while others are condemned as "wrong" for the family. The children are taught that by giving up their immediate desire for complete freedom of action for themselves, they gain the long-term security and caring protection of the family environment for the benefit of all.
     b. Ethics are based on a rational understanding of the need for a specific standard of conduct, as well as a deeply felt desire to follow the standard. Ethics function as a system of strongly held values for groups or individuals.
  2. **A "land ethic":** Those who value wilderness and the wilderness experience extend the notion of community to include the land and other life forms. The "land ethic" asserts that "a thing is right when it tends to preserve the integrity, stability, and beauty of the biotic community. It is wrong when it tends to do otherwise." (Leopold, 1966, p. 222) "...a land ethic changes the role of homo sapiens from conqueror of the land-community to plain member and citizen of it. It implies respect for his fellow-members, and also respect for the community as such" (Leopold, 1966, p. 204).

D. Implications of the "Land Ethic"
   1. **As professional wilderness education practitioners**
      a. Professional ethics are a code of conduct governing the actions of those working in a particular field of employment. Professional ethics are designed to encourage a standard level of acceptable performance by practitioners.
         (1) Professional ethics benefit clients by providing them a standard by which to evaluate the performance of individual practitioners. They allow the public to have a general level of confidence in the integrity of the profession.
         (2) Professional ethics benefit practitioners by providing them with established standards which can serve as guides during times of difficult decision making. They help individual practitioners to know what other professionals in the field would do in a situation, if faced with similar circumstances.
      b. What are the responsibilities of outdoor professionals to model behavior in keeping with the "land ethic"?
   2. **As members of our local community**
      a. Does our behavior as individuals and as a family make a difference with regard to the quality of life in our community?
      b. Should our belief in the "land ethic" influence our individual and family behavior in our home community?
      c. Does our belief in the "land ethic" imply a responsibility to educate or influence others in our community to share our belief?
      d. Does our belief in the "land ethic" imply a responsibility to influence community decision making insofar as it impacts upon the land?
   3. **As members of our nations/states**
      a. Does our behavior as citizens of our state or nation make a difference with regard to the quality of life in either?
      b. Should our belief in the "land ethic" influence our behavior as citizens of our state and nation?

c.   Does our belief in the "land ethic" imply a responsibility to act politically to influence state and national policies which have an impact on the land?

4. **As humans on this planet**

    a.   Does our behavior as human beings on this planet make a difference with regard to the quality of life on it?

    b.   Should our belief in the "land ethic" influence our behavior as it relates to all other living things on the planet?

IV. **INSTRUCTIONAL STRATEGIES & MATERIALS:**

  A. **Timing**

    1.   This topic incorporates virtually all of the unique aspects of the WEA curriculum. As such, it is impossible to deal with this topic in the context of a traditional class. All of the issues embraced by this topic must be addressed on a daily basis as the course progresses.

    2.   It is important to recognize that the objectives of this "lesson" go well beyond directing participants toward a specific set of backcountry conservation practices. By definition, the development of an environmental ethic suggests that participants will come to adopt a set of values which will be transferable to situations outside those of the immediate wilderness experience. To this end, instructors must be constantly aware of opportunities to help students recognize the broader implications of their backcountry behavior and assist them in understanding the need to establish a set of personal environmental standards that they can use in later life.

    3.   The following sequence is suggested for creating opportunities for instruction/reflection on backcountry ethics and conservation practices:

       a.   **Pre-course instruction**

           A presentation at the opening orientation of the course which identifies specific procedures to be followed in the backcountry and sets the standard for acceptable environmental behavior during the course.

       b.   **Teachable moments/formal class instruction**

Specific instruction concerning appropriate environmental behavior should be conducted as the opportunity or need arises throughout the course. (See specific lesson plans for additional teaching strategies.)

c. **Modeling**
Instructors must consistently model environmentally responsible behavior throughout the entire course.

d. **Processing of decision-making experiences**
During debriefings, campsite inspections, or in personal journals, participants should be encouraged to reflect upon those decision-making situations in which they have had to make choices regarding environmentally responsible conduct.

e. **Formal class on "Environmental Ethics and Backcountry Conservation Practices"**
This formal class should be conducted during the latter third of the course after students have had the chance to experience situations and behaviors which reflect a range of environmental responsibility.

B. **Strategies**
1. An understanding of ethics requires that a participant see a link between individual human action and the broader system of personal values which the action represents. To achieve this understanding, it is often advisable for instructors to begin by directing participant attention to concrete examples of behavior that may bear fruitful examination. Following are a few strategies for initiating this process:

a. Ask participants to describe in detail some incident during the expedition which they think illustrated either a very good or very poor example of environmentally responsible behavior.

b. Ask participants to create a short skit to be shown to the group which illustrates a conflict between responsible and irresponsible environmental behavior.

c. Write up a few short scenarios which involve conflict or choices between practices of varying degrees of environmental responsibility.

d. Create and then read an open-ended story in which a choice must be made between responsible and irresponsible environmental behavior. Ask students to role play a resolution to the problem in front of the group.

2. Once the concrete example has been examined, instructors should help participants "process" the experience. Instructors must establish a pattern of dialogue with the participants which closely resembles that used during a debriefing. In essence, the instructor should strive to help participants to move from a recognition of the significance of the specific behavior and its consequences, through a discussion of the values which the behavior reveals, to reach a general understanding of the need for a standard of environmental ethics. Once the participants understand the concept of personal environmental ethics, a discussion may ensue which explores the implications that such a code of ethics may have for one's behavior as a member of the local community, the state and nation, and finally, as a citizen of the world.

It should not be assumed that this transition from recognizing concrete circumstances to evaluating universal principles will occur in one class. Indeed, instructors should be laying the groundwork for this particular class from the very beginning of the course so that participants will have already discussed many of the incidents they now examine for the purpose of attaining a higher level of insight.

The diagram on the following page is designed to suggest the flow of dialogue that might attend this class

Environmental Ethics: A Progression

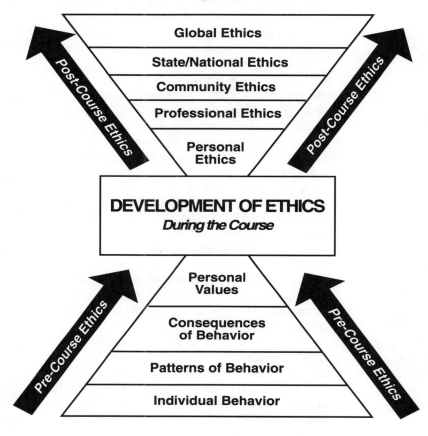

The lower pyramid or triangle represents development of ethics within oneself. The box containing the words "Development of Ethics" represents the content of this lesson and its application throughout the WEA course. Ideally, participants will start applying these ethics to the "outside" or larger world (i.e., to a broader context). The upper pyramid represents the application and synthesis of these newly developed ethics.

6. Expedition Behavior

I. **GOAL**: To have participants be aware of and practice good expedition behavior.

II. **OBJECTIVES**:
   A. Participants will be able to define expedition behavior.
   B. Participants will be able to list steps an individual can take to promote good expedition behavior.
   C. Participants will be able to explain the role expedition behavior plays in successful expeditions.
   D. Participants will be able to list the interrelationships involved in good expedition behavior.
   E. Participants will be able to list and explain components of conflict resolution.

III. **CONTENT**:
   A. Many believe that good expedition behavior is just one of four critical areas which lead to a successful expedition. **The four critical areas are:**
      1. Proper pre-trip planning
      2. Good expedition behavior
      3. Good leadership & quality decision-making skills
      4. Good outdoor skills

   B. **Definition**
      1. "Good expedition behavior is an awareness of the relationships..." which exist in the out-of-doors plus "...the motivation and character to be as concerned for others as one is for oneself." (Petzoldt, 1984, p. 168).
      2. Poor expedition behavior is characterized by, "a breakdown in human relations caused by selfishness, rationalization, ignorance of personal faults, dodging blame or responsibility, physical weakness and in extreme cases, not being able to risk one's

© 1992
The Wilderness Education Association
P.O. Box 89
Saranac Lake, New York 12983
(518) 891-2915 ext. 254

own survival to insure that of a companion."
(Petzoldt, 1984, p. 168).

C. **Consequences of Poor Expedition Behavior**
 1. Group members won't enjoy the expedition.
 2. Group objectives won't be met.
 3. Friendships may be lost.
 4. Individual safety may be compromised.

D. **Promoting Good Expedition Behavior**
 1. **Setting the tone**
 Setting a tone before a trip starts is critical to the success of a trip.
  a. The key to setting a tone is communication. One must communicate many things, including those listed below. The following is adapted from correspondence received by members of a 1971 expedition up Mt. McKinley (Petzoldt, 1984):
   (1) The group objectives: There must be an understanding and consensus on the group goals and objectives. It is important to agree on the priorities and what will happen if the objectives cannot be met.
   (2) Expectations: How group members can expect the trip to be conducted. These things might be considered "trip policy." For example:
    (a) Hiking – Learn to hike using rhythmic breathing to prevent fatigue and prevent exhaustion.
    (b) Short days – Everyone will go slowly to acclimate and prevent exhaustion. Camp will be set up early to allow time for healthy nutritious meals.
    (c) Eat well – Realize that diet affects attitude as well as strength.
    (d) Everyone does not have to do the same amount of work. Individuals should work to their capabilities. Work hard on good days, do less on others.
    (e) Sun – Watch out for the sun — it drains energy and sunburn can be crippling.

(f) Control body temperature – Try not to be too hot or too cold. Do what is necessary to keep the body temperature constant.

(g) Water – Drink lots of liquids. Water loss can be extreme and must be replaced.

(h) Sleep well – Being well rested contributes to getting along well with others.

(3) Additional policies may need to be determined relating to things such as:

(a) Feelings towards others

(b) Respecting opinions

(c) Proselytizing

(d) Relations between participants

(e) Relations between staff

(f) Relations between staff and participants

(g) Nudity

(h) Sexist attitudes

2. **Individual contributions to good expedition behavior**
As individuals, we contribute to good expedition behavior by keeping the following in mind:

a. Be tolerant and considerate of others.

b. Manage conflict effectively.

c. Maintain good personal hygiene practices. This is important for:

(1) Good health

(2) Aesthetics (who wants to look at someone with granola in their beard?)

d. Don't take offense

e. Maintain a "cow-like" attitude — have fun, don't let things become a hassle, there is no crisis.

f. Switch tent partners if there is no way to get along.

E. **Expedition Behavior Interrelationships**

1. **Individual to individual:** This relationship is personified by tent partners but exists between every individual in the group. Getting along with individuals can be accomplished by using the guidelines above.

2. **Individual to group:** The responsibility the individual has to be part of the group:

(1) Be organized.

(2) Be reasonably clean and neat.

(3) Be conscious of offensive and annoying habits.

(4) Be cooperative.

(5) Avoid dangerous activities.

(6) Take part in group activities.

(7) Be honest about personal needs (e.g., stop the group to take care of a blister).

3. **Group to individual:** The responsibility the group has to each individual. The group must accept the individual as a member of the group and keep from either ganging up on the individual or holding grudges against the individual.

4. **Group to group:**

a. The responsibility of groups to respect each other. When encountering other groups, it is best to be courteous but leave the group to its own privacy. Except in an emergency, it is best not to impose on other groups (e.g., borrowing or using food or equipment).

b. When encountering uneducated campers who are doing unsafe or harmful things to the environment, one must use tact and a soft sell educational approach. If an approach of assertiveness or arrogance is used, the objective of changing their behavior may be negated; they may resent being told what to do by strangers.

5. **Individual and group to multiple users:** Understanding that everyone has a right to use the out-of-doors within the limitations of the law is an important concept. Just because the group does not like a certain outdoor activity does not mean that the activity shouldn't be allowed. Respect of the multiple user will contribute to a better understanding of outdoor users and promote good public relations between groups.

6. **Individual and group to administrative agencies:** Understanding and respecting administrative agencies and their representatives contributes to good relations. Administrative representatives are generally hard-working professionals working for underfunded agencies. Their job is made easier when groups cooperate and work with them.

a. Obey rules and regulations. Don't ask for special favors which must be denied.

    b. Be courteous and cooperative when encountering rangers and other administrative representatives in the field.

    c. Sign in and out at registration locations as appropriate.

    d. Do not expect field representatives to know everything about the out-of-doors or the area they are responsible for. Employees of administrative agencies are rarely trained in the outdoors and are frequently transferred providing little time to become experts in their areas.

7. **Individual and group to the local populace:** Local residents of popular outdoor recreation areas often see visiting outdoor users as overeducated urban intruders. They are sometimes politically threatened by these outsiders. Every effort should be made by outdoor users to understand their point of view and try to be cooperative and respectful.

F. **Conflict and Its Resolution**

Conflict is a natural stage of group development and its effective management is essential for successful group evolution. Listed below are stages of defining and resolving group conflict based on Johnson & Johnson (1987).

1. Define the conflict.
2. Confront the individual(s).
    a. Negotiate
    b. Openly communicate feelings in minimally threatening ways.
    c. Try to understand the other person's views.
    d. Don't demand change.
3. Agree on the definition of the conflict.
4. Communicate position and feelings.
5. Communicate cooperative intentions.
6. Take the other's perspective.
7. Reach agreement through negotiation.

IV. **INSTRUCTIONAL STRATEGIES & MATERIALS:**

A. **Timing**

It is important to set a tone early in the trip and cover certain aspects of expedition behavior informally or by using teachable moments.

1.   A formal exercise or discussion helping to set group norms is essential early in the trip.
2.   A formal class on expedition behavior can be taught later in the trip and reinforced with examples which have occurred during the trip. Examples are critical to bring this topic from the abstract to reality.
3.   The topic of conflict resolution can be explored at the following times:
     a.   Early in the trip so that the skills can be used in situations that emerge.
     b.   At the time of conflict so participants' need to know is maximized.

B.   **Strategies**
     Skits can be used very effectively to demonstrate the points being made.

C.   **Activities**
     1.   Skits
          a.   On pieces of paper, write down incidents relating to expedition behavior observed during the trip. Set the incidents in different frameworks so they are not obvious to participants and will not embarrass or offend group members.
          b.   Select small groups to reenact these scenes and then discuss how they fit into the topic of expedition behavior. When selecting the groups to do skits, avoid selecting individuals involved in the particular incidents to reenact "their" incident. There is a better chance for them to "get the message" if they can observe the skit that relates to them.
          c.   Discussion of the skit and its application to the group allows for carry over and reinforcement.
     2.   Readings: Read aloud or assign readings related to expedition behavior such as "Ordeal on Everest" by Murray Sayle, in LIFE Magazine, July 2, 1971.
     3.   Conflict resolution can be taught by having the group "invent" conflicts in pairs and role play the resolution in front of the group.

7. Fire Site Preparation and Care

I. **GOAL**: To have participants prepare, care for, and return a fire site to its natural state.

II. **OBJECTIVES**:
   A. Participants will be able to list environmental considerations in selecting a site for a fire.
   B. Participants will be able to list and explain the considerations in determining whether a fire should be built or a backpacking stove should be used.
   C. Participants will be able to explain the function and rationale for using a fire.
   D. Participants will be able to distinguish between the three basic soil types and explain their role in fire site preparation.
   E. Participants will be able to demonstrate and explain how to prepare three types of sites for fires.
   F. Participants will be able to list and explain safety considerations in selecting a site for a fire.
   G. Participants will be able to demonstrate the proper means of site restoration.

III. **CONTENT**:
   A. **Environmental Considerations**
       1. Considerations in using a fire rather than a stove.
           a. **Fires should only be used when:**
               (1) There is an ample supply of dead wood on the ground.
               (2) Wood used will be naturally replenished within a reasonable time.
               (3) There is a safe location for a fire.
               (4) There is little or no potential for adverse environmental impact.
               (5) They are permitted by law.

b. Except in an emergency, fires should be considered luxuries and not true necessities.

2. **Site selection considerations**

   a. **Sites may be suitable if:**
      (1) The site is pristine and shows little or no sign of human use.
      (2) There is little chance that it will be used again before the site has a chance to recover.
      (3) The site is heavily impacted and use will not appreciably impact it more.
      (4) There is no evidence of erosion and/or minimal potential for erosion to occur.
      (5) An existing safe fireplace exists, in which case it should be used.

   c. **Locations to avoid include:**
      (1) Low-impact campsites which, with increased use, might become high-impact campsites.
      (2) Biologically sensitive areas such as those with many roots or easily damaged vegetation.
      (3) Areas with large or waterlogged rocks that may explode or be blackened by the fire.

B. **Rationale for Fires**

   Fires play a special role in the history of humans as well as the history of modern wilderness travel. Fires play a role in both function and aesthetics. Although the negative impacts of fire are numerous, there is no reason why they cannot be used in many areas as long as judgment prevails.

C. **Functions of Fires**

   These functions are listed by priority. As environmental concerns increase, the function of the fire must be of a higher priority to justify its use.

   1. **Heat for emergency warmth and drying:** In an emergency situation, a fire could be a life saver. However, in most cases proper clothing and equipment help conserve the energy that good nutrition will provide.

   2. **Food preparation:** This is a traditional and valid purpose for a fire, assuming environmental conditions permit.

   3. **Aesthetic/psychological appeal:** This is another traditional purpose for a fire. Environmental

concerns in many parts of North America negate justification for fires based purely on aesthetic grounds.

4. **Heat for general warmth and drying:** Although heat is a pleasant by-product of a fire built for cooking or pleasure, it is difficult to justify it for warmth alone. Proper clothing, equipment, and good nutrition offer more sound alternatives to fires for comfort and warmth while in the outdoors.

D. **Soils**

There are three basic layers of soil to recognize when selecting a site for a fire. (This is an oversimplification of soil types. Judgment should be used in choosing a fire site that minimizes impact.)

1. **Litter**
    a. It is composed of leaves, twigs, and other natural organic matter.
    b. It is found on top of the ground.
    c. It is highly flammable. Care must be taken not to build a fire on top of, or next to, litter.

2. **Duff**
    a. Decomposing litter which may be compacted or compressed.
    b. Generally found under the litter but sometimes found on the surface, particularly where an area has been heavily camped and the litter has been trampled or picked clean for fires.
    c. It is flammable and burns slowly, usually without flame. Care must be taken not to build fires on duff, as duff fires can burn for days undetected until something more combustible is ignited.

3. **Mineral soil**
    a. Inorganic material made up of sand, gravel, and stones.
    b. Generally found under the duff, but sometimes found on or near the surface, particularly near streams and where trees have been uprooted.

E. **Safety Considerations**
1. **General considerations**
    The Boy Scouts of America discuss three factors of fire safety:

a. A safe location (which eliminates the need to reach over the fire)
b. A safe fire
c. Complete extinction of the fire

2. **Specific considerations**
    a. Wind direction
    b. Tending the fire. It is advisable to never leave a fire unattended!
    c. Distance from tents and other equipment
    d. Nearby combustible materials (roots, grasses, trees, duff)
    e. Available water
    f. Weather conditions (drought)

F. **Sites**
    1. **Established fireplaces**
        If an established fireplace exists, it should be used. Preparing alternate sites will increase impact in an already impacted area.
    2. **Existing informal fire rings**
        a. In heavily camped areas, one or more fire rings may be found.
        b. If a fire ring exists, it should be used as long as it is safe. If the site is not safe, it is better not to have any fire than create more impact within the area.
        c. If more than one fire ring exists in a campsite, it is advisable to leave a well-placed and clean one for others to use and then dismantle and reclaim the others. Always leave one in a high-impact site. Otherwise, they may be built again in a more undesirable location (Hampton & Cole, 1988).
    3. **Mound or pedestal fires**
        Constructed with a layer of mineral soil collected from streambeds, uprooted trees, or other areas of exposed mineral soil.
        a. Spread at least three inches (8 cm.) of soil over an appropriate base such as a boulder or other area where the heat generated from the fire will not injure plant or animal life in the soil below. If necessary, collect any litter or other readily combustible material away from the site to save for restoring the site later.

b.   Insure that the area is larger than the anticipated fire (approximately two feet square, or 30 cm.).

c.   The site is now ready to build a fire.

4. **Fire pan technique**

This is made the same way as a mound fire except that it is built on an artificial, non-flammable surface which further reduces the fire's impact and aids in restoration. (A good fire pan can be made from a 3 x 3 foot section of an old Forest Service fire shelter.)

5. **Firepits**

These are constructed by digging a hole into the mineral layer of soil.

a.   Collect all litter from the site and store it for restoring the site later.

b.   Dig out a square or circle of sod large enough for a fire, approximately 18"-24" (45-61 cm.).

(1)   Store it where it won't get trampled.

(2)   Water it if necessary to maintain the vegetation growing in it.

c.   Remove any remaining duff (if there is no mineral soil within eight inches, restore the site and look for an alternative one).

d.   Line the sides with mineral soil.

e.   The site is now ready for building a fire.

G. **Site Restoration**

The process of restoring the site to its natural condition before camp is broken to make it look as if there had been no fire there.

1. **Considerations before restoring the site**

a.   Be sure to burn the wood to ash, minimizing large chunks or burnt wood which will be difficult to restore.

b.   Put the fire out the night before breaking camp. Cook on a stove the next morning.

2. **Restoring the site**

a.   Make sure the fire is completely out by dousing with water and stirring until it is cool enough to touch with bare hands.

b.   Distribute the ashes randomly through the woods.

c.   If more wood than necessary was collected, scatter it through the woods.

d.   If a mound fire was used, replace the mineral soil to its original location.

e.   If a firepit was used, replace the soil in the same order that it was removed, taking care to restore the litter layer and blending it in with the surrounding area. Water the sod well.

    f.   The major problem with firepit restoration is their tendency to sink and form a shallow but noticeable depression in the surface. This can be corrected by stamping the mineral soil before the sod is replaced and/or leaving the sod plug slightly raised to allow for settling.

IV. INSTRUCTIONAL STRATEGIES & MATERIALS:

A. Timing
This lesson is best taught early in the course, although the timing may be determined by the fire-building regulations of the course area.

B. Strategies
This lesson lends itself nicely to student instruction and works effectively if combined with "Frying and Baking" and "Fire Building."

C. Materials
1. A suitable site for building a fire
2. Shovel

8. Fire Building

I. **GOAL**: To have participants build a safe, functional, and environmentally-sound fire.

II. **OBJECTIVES**:
A. Participants will be able to identify and select appropriate wood for the construction of a fire.
B. Participants will be able to list the three common components of fire and understand their role in fire building.
C. Participants will be able to list and explain the function of the common materials used in fire construction.
D. Participants will be able to list safety considerations in fire construction.
E. Participants will be able to demonstrate a minimum of one way to build and light a fire.
F. Participants will be able to list considerations in starting a fire during inclement weather.
G. Participants will be able to demonstrate and explain environmental considerations in the selection of fuel, and the construction, use, and care of the fire.
H. Participants will be able to demonstrate and explain considerations in igniting the fire.

III. **CONTENT**:
A. **Safety Considerations**
    1. If necessary, review safety considerations from the "Fire Site Preparation and Care" lesson.
    2. If necessary, review safety considerations from the "Introductory Cooking" lesson.
    3. Some major safety considerations to reinforce are:
        a. Make sure there is a ready source of water available to put the fire out in the event of an emergency.

© 1992
The Wilderness Education Association
P.O. Box 89
Saranac Lake, New York 12983
(518) 891-2915 ext. 254

b.   Wear gloves around the fire to prevent burning and/or drying out hands.

c.   Never leave a fire unattended for more than a very short time.

B.   **Environmental Considerations**
1.   If necessary, review environmental considerations in the "Fire Site Preparation and Care" lesson.
2.   Some major considerations to reinforce are:
a.   If in doubt, use a stove.
b.   Only collect wood that is already down on the ground.

C.   **Identifying and Selecting Firewood**
1.   The selection of firewood is generally a function of availability. Use what is legally available. In most regions of the country, there isn't a lot of choice. Ideally, one would select firewood based on the following considerations:
a.   **Softwoods** (e.g., pine, spruce, and cedar) are convenient for use as tinder and kindling. They ignite readily and burn hot.
b.   **Hardwoods** (e.g., maple, yellow birch, and black cherry) are excellent for obtaining hot long lasting coals, providing a steady temperature for cooking and baking.
2.   It has been determined that fires will only be used when there is an ample supply of firewood on the ground and the wood burned will be naturally replenished in a reasonable time. (See "Fire Site Preparation and Care" lesson.)
3.   Firewood selection should be based on the following considerations:
a.   Only collect wood that is already down. Remember..."rules are for fools." In rainy weather, when a fire is necessary, one might pick the fine, dead tinder which is still attached in the undergrowth of a conifer.
b.   Collect enough wood to maintain the fire (usually twice as much as originally estimated). Few things are as frustrating as having to run off and collect firewood once the fire is started.
c.   Collect wood of different sizes (less than the size of a matchstick up to three inches in

diameter) and stack the wood according to size.
This provides convenient access to wood as the
fire is started.

D. **The Three Common Components of Fire**
There must be a balance of fuel, heat, and oxygen to have
a successful fire. When having difficulty starting a fire, it
is often helpful to think of which component is out of
balance and try to establish the proper balance.
1.   **Fuel**: Wood provides the fuel in campfires. The key
is to have the correct size fuel for the amount of heat
available. Fuel the size of 4" logs, with heat generated from fuel the size of matchsticks, won't work.
2.   **Heat**: Heat ignites the fuel and must be balanced
with it. Large fuel will not ignite until the heat of the
fire rises to a suitable temperature to thoroughly
heat the wood. Water vapor is often profuse next to
the ground and will inhibit combustion. The fire
should be ignited a few inches above ground level.
3.   **Oxygen**: There must be room for oxygen. Allow for
ample air circulation and arrange the fuel so that
oxygen can get to the fire.

E.   **Materials In Fire Construction**
1.   **Tinder**
a.   Fine, flammable material which will ignite from
the heat of a match.
b.   Birch bark (collected from the ground), pine, or
spruce pitch, and fine twigs (twiggies).
c.   If the group must depend on fires, it is
important to have a plastic bag of these
materials for a rainy day.
2.   **Kindling**
a.   Small diameter branches (3/4" or less) or split
wood which ignites from the heat of the
burning tinder and, in turn, provides the heat
to ignite the larger fuel.
b.   Softwoods such as pine, spruce, and cedar are
very suitable for kindling. They ignite readily
and give off plenty of heat to ignite larger fuels.
3.   **Fuel**
a.   Firewood which provides coals and uniform
heat for cooking.

b.   Hardwoods such as maple, hickory, and apple do an admirable job of providing good coals for cooking.

F.   **Laying the Fire**

   1.   Everyone has a favorite way to lay a fire. How it is laid is not as important as how well it functions. Does the lay of the fire allow for the proper balance of the three elements necessary for a good fire?

   2.   When using a firepit, or if the ground is particularly cold or moist, it is helpful to lay a row of logs, bark, or other material on the ground before the fire is laid. This insulates the fire from cold and moisture and allows the heat to be used for combustion, rather than absorbed by the ground.

   3.   Lay the smallest, most combustible material at the bottom. As heat rises, this will allow for the most efficient use of available heat.

   4.   Several types of fires are listed below.

      a.   **Lean-to**

         By providing a bed of tinder and leaning tinder and kindling against a "lean-to support" or larger piece of kindling, an efficient fire can often be quickly built.

      b.   **Tepee**

         (1)   By building a tepee of kindling around an abundant supply of tinder, a healthy fire can eventually grow by gradually increasing the size of the outermost wood.

         (2)   At some point, the tepee will collapse from its own weight. The challenge is not to let it collapse until the fire is large enough to sustain itself.

         (3)   A tepee fire is one of the most effective lays in rainy weather, allowing the outer wood to dry while the inner tinder and kindling is burning.

         (4)   To keep the tepee going until the outer wood ignites, continue replacing tinder and kindling as it burns.

   c. **Log cabin**
A series of logs are criss-crossed log-cabin style, allowing for plenty of oxygen and a place to carefully set cooking pots.

G. **Inclement Weather Suggestions**
1. Use your twiggy bag (a bag of twiggies, birch bark, pitch, and other tinders collected on a sunny day and saved for a rainy day).
2. Oozing pitch from coniferous trees ignites under the most adverse conditions. Carefully scrape pitch from the tree, trying not to injure the bark.
3. Look for dry tinder under logs, boulders, at the base of large trees, and other dry areas.
4. Carve dry wood out of the core of wet kindling.
5. Build a tepee fire, being sure to keep the center well stoked.

H. **Lighting the Fire**
1. Don't be afraid to use paper if it's available.
2. Remember that heat rises, so when striking a match, try to hold the lit end lower than the rest of the match. This will allow the match to stay lit and burn hotter.
3. Light the fire upwind so the heat generated will be blown towards the fire and not away from it.
4. Homemade or commercial firestarters made from paraffin and paper can be carried for lighting fires in moist or emergency conditions.

IV. **INSTRUCTIONAL STRATEGIES & MATERIALS:**
A. **Timing**
Depending on whether stoves are used extensively or not, this class can be taught as needed and in conjunction with the "Fire Site Preparation and Care" lesson.

B. **Strategies**
1. This class lends itself nicely to student teaching.
2. Many instructors use a lecture/demonstration format followed by participant practice of the skill.

C. **Materials**
1. Fuel
2. Matches
3. Cotton gloves
4. Shovel
5. Water

9. Group Processing and Debriefing

I. **GOAL**: Participants will be able to demonstrate an ability to organize and conduct effective briefing, debriefing, and processing sessions.

II. **OBJECTIVES**:
  A. Participants will be able to describe the purpose of a WEA debriefing.
  B. Participants will be able to describe the major considerations in organizing daily briefing and debriefing sessions.
  C. Participants will be able to describe the major components of successful briefing and debriefing sessions.
  D. Participants will be able to explain the purpose of the "processing" component of the debriefing.
  E. Participants will be able to conduct successful briefings and debriefings in the field.

III. **CONTENT**:
  A. **Group Processing is Critical to the WEA Curriculum**
      It is one of the most important evaluation tools in developing judgment. Participants can analyze and evaluate experiences and learn from each others' successes and failures.

  B. **Organizing the Session**
      Many of the basic considerations for organizing a briefing or debriefing are identical to those involved in setting up a formal class presentation. See "Teaching Techniques" lesson for more detail.
      1. **Timing the session**
          a. The session is best conducted at a regular time each day so that it becomes an established, integral part of the daily camp routine.

The Wilderness Education Association
P.O. Box 89
Saranac Lake, New York 12983
(518) 891-2915 ext. 254

b. Early morning is often a good time, since participants should be alert and previous day's activities will still be relatively fresh in their memories.

c. Should an early morning campsite move be necessary, the session can be held along the trail during an extended break. This is preferable to skipping the daily session entirely or trying to hold it after a long day of travel when participants are tired.

2. **Location of the session**

a. The session site should be located in an area sheltered from the elements and away from any distractions.

b. The meeting should be located away from areas of high traffic use within the campsite (i.e., cooking areas) to minimize human impact on any given area.

c. The meeting site should be large enough to accommodate all participants comfortably.

3. **Preparing for the session**

a. All participants should know the time and location of the day's briefing/debriefing site well in advance. LOD's can inform each set of tent partners during wake-up call.

b. All participants should be informed or reminded of the routine.
   (1) Appropriate clothing
   (2) Notebook and pencil
   (3) Insulation pad for sitting

c. Participants should be reminded of any special materials they will need to bring to the session.
   (1) Maps and compasses
   (2) Resource books
   (3) Special reports (e.g., logger's notes, etc.)
   (4) Journals

d. All participants who may have to make presentations or reports during the session should be reminded of their responsibilities so they can be organized and ready.

e. Participants should be discouraged from bringing food or drinks to the session, as they are distracting. In addition, participants who

worked hard to get their meals completed
before the meeting often resent the inefficiency
of others.

f.   Punctuality for all group activities is an issue
which must be addressed early in the course.
Efficiency should be balanced with enjoyment
and a non-stressful atmosphere.

C.   **Planning the Session**
The LOD should have a clear idea of the general
components of the sessions, as well as a specific set of
objectives to be met during the session.

1.   **Components of the session**
In general, all sessions are comprised of three broad
components, each with its own essential function.
Although the order in which these components are
addressed may differ, they all should appear in
virtually every meeting.

a.   **Informational component**
Each session should include the information
participants will need to prepare and plan
adequately for the day's activities, and for any
future events that may require pre-planning.

(1)   A specific itinerary for the day should be
announced. This should include times,
location of specific classes, moving of
camp, etc.

(2)   Assignments for the day: The LOD should
make and announce all special assign-
ments/tasks for the day (e.g., sweep, logger,
scout, nature-of-the-day, etc.) so participants
can be prepared for their tasks.

(3)   Classes for the day: Participants responsible for making special presentations
during the day should be reminded of
their assignments.

b.   **Logistical component**
Most sessions include an opportunity for group
participation in the detailed planning of day
trips, moving camp, travel routes, etc.

(1)   Participants can discuss and select the best
routes, identify significant topographic
features, estimate bearings, and write out
time control plans.

(2) Participants can discuss individual and group gear to be taken on a trip and determine who will carry them.

(3) If the group is splitting up for the day's travel, participants can discuss the objectives of the trip and the route, apportion group gear, determine group membership, and submit written emergency evacuation plans.

c. **Educational component**
One of the most important functions of a debriefing session is the opportunity for group members to share and process their experiences.

(1) All sessions should include a quick survey of the mental and physical status of each participant.

(a) All expedition members should know how others are feeling mentally and physically, so that group plans and activities may take this into account.

(b) Participants should recognize the session as an appropriate arena for airing personal views and settling interpersonal differences. An atmosphere of objective openness, tolerance, and compassion must be maintained at all sessions so that group members feel comfortable expressing their thoughts and feelings.

(2) Sessions should include an analysis and evaluation of the various decision-making opportunities of the previous day. This particular aspect of the session is absolutely crucial to the development of effective decision-making skills. This "processing" phase of the session requires a high degree of skill, and therefore requires discipline in preparing and guiding the discussion. (See D. 2. in this chapter for more detail on processing.)

D. **Conducting Sessions**
1. **General guidelines and suggestions**
a. Proper technical and mental preparation are essential for a successful session. Refer to the

"Teaching Techniques" lesson to review aspects of communication that may prove helpful in conducting an effective session.

b. A small notepad with brief reminders of important information or topics is very useful for reference during the session.

c. Writing out specific objectives beforehand helps to focus the leader's attention on what must be done and will help clarify what is or is not relevant discussion during the meeting.

d. Keep the session "moving" by insisting that participants focus on the issues at hand and refrain from clearly unnecessary banter or inappropriate comments. Don't be timid about diplomatically curtailing a rambling discussion. If necessary, designate a "taskmaster" to keep the discussion focused.

e. To maintain group attention, allow time for stretching or bathroom breaks.

f. Above all else, be "professional" in presentation and demeanor. A good-humored but essentially business-like approach to the session will set an appropriate educational tone.

2. **The "processing" component:** considerations for leading the analysis/evaluation phase of the session.

a. Fundamental to the development of decision-making skills is an ability to "process" experience (i.e., an ability to reflect on, describe, analyze, and communicate in some way, that which was recently experienced). The analysis/evaluation phase of each debriefing is an opportunity for each participant to process the previous day's experience and share in the evaluative judgments which come out of the discussion (Quinsland & Ginkel, 1984).

b. If all participants are to process their own experiences successfully, they all must take part in the discussion concerning the previous day's experience. The individual who leads the discussion should be aware of the skills and techniques necessary for leading an effective group discussion. For more detailed suggestions on leading a discussion, see the "Teaching Techniques" lesson.

c. "Processing" should begin with a brief, chronological recounting of the previous day's activities. This helps refresh memories for journal writing, allows the group to develop a common interpretation of the shared experience which may bind the group together, and identifies those moments of decision-making, crisis, or conflict which need to be explored.

d. Once the previous day's events have been established, the process of analyzing those events may proceed.

    (1) Participants should be encouraged to specifically identify those moments when significant decision-making situations arose. As these moments are identified, the discussion leader should ask questions which focus on why each decision was made:

        (a) What factors influenced the decision?

        (b) What personal considerations had to be taken into account?

        (c) What possible options were open to the decision-makers? Who made the decision?

    (2) At this stage of the discussion, hasty conclusions about whether a decision was "good" or "bad" should be discouraged.

e. At some stage during the discussion, the decision-makers (frequently the LOD) should be invited to critique their own performance and explain the rationale for their actions. Decision-makers should be given an opportunity to fully explore and communicate their own interpretations of events before the group moves on to the evaluation stage.

f. Once the group understands the various factors that entered into the making of a specific decision and the decision-makers have had an opportunity to explore and explain the rationale for their actions, then the discussion leader should invite comments which are evaluative:

71

(1) Was the decision a good one?

    (2) In what other ways may the situation have been successfully handled?

    (3) What did you learn from this situation?

  g. Throughout the processing experience, it is important that the discussion leader try to keep the tone as constructive and positive as possible without sacrificing a truthful assessment of the decision-maker's strengths and weaknesses. Conflict and injured pride that come from group criticism are inevitable and, though unpleasant, are an essential aspect of the educational process that leads to the growth of quality decision-making.

  h. Good listening skills are essential to ensure that opinions are being heard and understood. Active and silent listening activities may be used if listening problems are encountered.

  i. At the conclusion of the processing discussion, it may be helpful for the discussion leader to summarize conclusions made by the group with some brief statements. This not only highlights the main points of the discussion, but also helps to de-personalize some of the criticism that may have been directed at one individual and helps turn the focus toward understandings which can benefit any leader.

IV. **INSTRUCTIONAL STRATEGIES & MATERIALS**:

 A. **Timing**

  Since briefing and debriefing sessions begin at the outset of the expedition, instruction in briefing and debriefing technique can begin immediately through an example set by instructors. Student LOD's may be expected to conduct all but the "processing" aspects of a debriefing by the third or fourth day of the expedition.

 B. **Strategies**

  1. Teaching briefing and debriefing through daily example seems to be one of the most effective means of helping participants learn this technique. As each discussion leader helps the group examine the briefing or debriefing style of the previous day's

leader, instructors should emphasize positive suggestions and ideas that are brought out.

2. It is generally a good idea for instructors to conduct sessions for the first few days of the expedition. This not only sets a good example for participants to follow, but also sets a tone of objective openness and candor when instructors lead the self-critical aspects and evaluation of their own performance. Participants will see that the ability to evaluate one's own strengths and weaknesses candidly is an essential element of quality leadership.

10. Group Development

by Chris Cashel Ed.D.

I. **GOAL**: To provide participants with a framework for understanding the stages of group growth.

II. **OBJECTIVES:**
   A. Participants will be able to identify the stages of group development.
   B. Participants will be able to identify behaviors in the group which are conducive to group development.
   C. Participants will be able to identify behaviors which are undesirable and interfere with group development.
   D. Participants will be aware of emotional issues which promote or detract from the group's ability to develop.
   E. Participants will be aware of the leader's role and responsibility in group development.

III. **CONTENT**:
   A. **Characteristics of a Group**
      Participants and assigned leaders make up the group. All group members have needs, expectations, skills, and emotions.
      1. Groups have both task functions (i.e., content, things to do) and maintenance functions (i.e., process, ways to keep in working order, interpersonal relations) to perform.
      2. The nature of the task and the experience of the group dictate the balance between task and maintenance functions.
      3. The leadership style used by the assigned leader in any stage or in any situation will affect the task/maintenance balance.

4. Group members will assume a variety of roles and behaviors to accommodate task and maintenance functions.

5. As roles and behaviors emerge from the group and are accepted, the group begins to take on a unique personality.

6. The process that moves a group from a collection of individuals to a productive, interactive group follows a pattern.

B. **Stages of Group Development**

1. **Orientation** (getting acquainted)
   Other terminology that parallels this stage: Dependency, Task Functions: Orientation (Jones, 1973); Forming (Schoel, Prouty, & Radcliffe, 1988)

   a. This stage is ambiguous for the participants. They may search for structure and test the leader. At this stage, the group can be described as a collection of individuals.

   b. The group is dependent on the leader.

   c. The leader's role:
      (1) Accept dependence and assume a stronger leadership style.
      (2) Set the tone and acceptable parameters of behavior.
      (3) Listen, smile, and support members.
      (4) Maintain an even keel.
      (5) Use humor.
      (6) Encourage introduction of group members.
      (7) Speak to the group as a whole about group issues. (Avoid giving one individual extra information prior to group knowledge.)
      (8) Limit information to the essentials.

2. **Conflict** (struggling forward)
   Other terminology that parallels this stage: Task Functions: Organization (Jones, 1973); Storming (Prouty, Schoel, & Radcliffe, 1988)

   a. Members are trying to organize themselves into roles.

   b. Members may show impatience with each other, especially less skilled or "different" members.

c.   Members may interrupt or disagree over plans or ideas. They are vying for attention and leadership within the group.

    d.   The leader's role:

       (1)   Support all members equally.

       (2)   Encourage group members to discuss and resolve conflicts.

       (3)   The leader should not think that she or he needs to "fix" all problems.

3.   **Integration or cohesion** (becoming personal)
Other terminology that parallels this stage:
Task Functions: Data-flow (Jones, 1973); Norming (Schoel, Prouty, & Radcliffe, 1988)

    a.   This is a period of reconciliation when members listen and seek consensus, accept differences, and are willing to compromise and work together to accomplish tasks.

    b.   The leader's role:

       (1)   Continue to support and praise positive behaviors.

       (2)   Involve the group in decisions and let consequences occur without compromising the safety of the group.

4.   **Achievement or interdependence** (working together)
Other terminology that parallels this stage:
Task Functions: Problem-solving (Jones, 1973); Performing (Schoel, Prouty, & Radcliffe, 1988)

    a.   The group is functional and interpersonal relationships are strong.

    b.   The group is efficient and capable of both task and maintenance functions. This is an ideal stage to reach. It is unlikely many groups will get this far, but they may experience moments in this stage.

    c.   The leader's role: Enjoyment and satisfaction.

5.   **Order (saying good-bye)**

    a.   Members are satisfied and unwilling to reassess norms or to introduce new ideas for consideration.

    b.   Apathy and a slower progress toward reaching new goals may occur.

c.   The group may reminisce about past group experiences as they prepare to separate.

    d.   Some individuals may withdraw.

    e.   The leader's role:

       (1) Provide feedback and encourage the accomplishment of new goals — finish strong!

       (2) If time allows, confront the group with a debriefing of the course and prepare them for re-entering society.

C. **Emotional Factors**

    1.   Emotional factors may affect the ability of the group to move from one stage to another.

    2.   Shutz's theory uses three emotional phases or levels that the group experiences.

    3.   The emotional or psychological phases are cyclical and continuous, and emotional needs in each phase must be satisfied before moving on. The phases coincide with the group's development and the degree to which members feel part of the group.

      a. **Inclusion**: People wonder if they fit in and have appropriate skills to help the group meet goals, or if they will be accepted. This is an early issue which may reoccur with each new situation.

        (1) **Signs of when inclusion is adequate:**

          (a) Individual needs are recognized and accepted.

          (b) Participation is evenly distributed among members.

          (c) There is good interaction.

          (d) The group can articulate goals and is committed to their goals.

        (2) **Signs of when inclusion is inadequate:**

          (a) Members may be late to meetings

          (b) Some members may feel excluded.

          (c) There is little interaction and participation is unevenly distributed.

          (d) An overall lack of confidence is observable in the group.

          (e) There is a lack of cooperation.

          (f) Individual (versus group) behaviors and decisions are evident.

      b. **Control**: There are feelings about roles, responsibility, and power — who has it and who wants it. Control issues reflect each person's feelings of where power is in a group. They also reflect one's own feeling of competence in any given circumstance.

(1) **Signs of when control is adequate:**
   (a) The decision-making process is clear.
   (b) Conflict is accepted and dealt with.
   (c) There is shared leadership and power.
   (d) There is bargaining within the group.
   (e) The group is productive.

(2) **Signs of when control is inadequate:**
   (a) The group uses poor decision-making processes.
   (b) There are power struggles.
   (c) There is a lack of leadership.
   (d) There is criticism and competitiveness within the group.
   (e) The instructor may resort to using a more definite structure and imposing decisions.

c. **Affection**: liking others and being liked.

(1) **Signs of when affection is adequate:**
   (a) Communication is open and honest.
   (b) Feelings are expressed.
   (c) Group members feel free to be different and still be accepted.
   (d) Group members are receptive to new ideas.
   (e) Group members feel close to one another.

(2) **Signs of when affection is inadequate:**
   (a) There is limited communication.
   (b) Members withhold feedback.
   (c) There is a lack of trust of others.
   (d) There is dissatisfaction with the group.

3. As these cyclical stages are repeated, ideas and feelings are also repeated and deepened.

4. Everyone, including instructors, experience emotional stages of feeling adequate, liked, and competent. It is important to give enough information and enough responsibility for the group to establish bonds to keep it functioning.

D. **Leadership Skills That Enhance Group Development**
1. Set a tone early. Encourage consistent behaviors and a "cow-like" attitude.
2. Communicate through listening, feedback, and constructive criticism.
3. Use the decision-making process.
4. Use conflict resolution techniques.
5. Explain group dynamics within the framework of expedition behavior. This allows for either success or failure of goal accomplishment.
6. Use an appropriate leadership style for the developmental phase of the group.
7. Allow for group maintenance (e.g., clarify ideas, evaluate suggestions, diagnose problems, etc.).

IV. **INSTRUCTIONAL STRATEGIES & MATERIALS:**
A. **Timing**
Certainly a fitting time to address group development is when the group has reached a storming stage.

B. **Strategies**
Using their own group as an example (or another group of which they have been a member), ask participants to name situations that illustrate different stages of group development.

11. Latrine Construction and Use

I. **GOAL**: To have participants learn and practice techniques of waste disposal with safety and minimum environmental impact.

II. **OBJECTIVES**:
   A. Participants will be able to list the considerations in constructing a latrine.
   B. Participants will know the physical, environmental, and aesthetic consequences of not properly disposing of human waste.
   C. Participants will be able to construct a latrine.
   D. Participants will be able to use a cathole.
   E. Participants will be able to use a latrine.
   F. Participants will be able to close a latrine.

III. **CONTENT**:
   A. **Consequences of not properly disposing of waste**
   Many campers can tell stories of their experiences finding human waste in strange and disgusting places with no consideration for aesthetic or environmental consequences. Human waste has been seen in the middle of the trail, on rocks in the middle of streams, and even in the crotch of a tree four feet off the ground! Humans are generally animals of convenience, and unless the impact of these actions is understood, change is unlikely.
   1. **Aesthetic impact**
      Aesthetics is the study of beauty. Someone who leaves human waste in visible sight of others is insensitive to beauty and inconsiderate of other users. Wilderness users must make an effort to preserve the beauty of the outdoors.

© 1992
The Wilderness Education Association
P.O. Box 89
Saranac Lake, New York 12983
(518) 891-2915 ext. 254

2. **Physical impact**
   a. Human waste has the potential to affect water sources profoundly by contributing to waterborne diseases such as giardia, cholera, typhoid fever, and other similar diseases.
   b. A variety of illnesses caused by human contamination have been documented in wilderness waters. The most prevalent – giardiasis – is caused by a protozoan. Its symptoms are severe diarrhea, stomach cramps, and nausea. Proper disposal of human waste helps to minimize the spread of this disease.

3. **Environmental impact**
   The presence of fecal bacteria in water systems is an indicator of contamination. Other animals such as coyotes, bighorn sheep, beaver, and cattle may also be affected by water-borne organisms.

B. **Considerations in Latrine Construction**
   Constructing a latrine requires a balance of various needs.
   1. **No two latrines will ever be the same**
      Individuals should strive to be creative while meeting the needs listed below. It may help to remember the first letter of each consideration as the "three P's and a D" in latrine construction.
      a. **Pollution**
         Make sure all latrines are located at least 150 feet from water sources and in well-drained soil. They should not be located in an area which may be flooded during wet weather.
      b. **Depth**
         (1) Latrines should be dug at a depth where good biological action will help break down waste. Biological action means that bacteria, insects, and other animal life will help decompose waste. In most environments, the duff layer provides the best depth (8-16"/20-40 cm. maximum) for latrines. (See the "Fire Site Preparation and Care" lesson for a discussion of soil layers, if necessary.)
         (2) Although it is important to keep latrines relatively shallow in order to promote waste decay, it is also important that

latrines are deep enough to prevent animals from digging them up. This problem varies with course locations and special environments.

   c. **Privacy**

      Our society has conditioned us to desire privacy in disposing of our waste. If privacy is not provided, group members are likely to not use the latrine and to leave their waste randomly in the woods with little or no concern for the environment.

   d. **Proximity**

      While privacy must be maintained, it is just as important to make sure latrines are close enough to the campsite for group members to use. If they are too far away and not convenient to use, group members are once again more likely to leave their waste randomly in the woods.

2. **Latrine construction**

   a. Using the previously discussed considerations, find a location.

     (1) Try to pick a comfortable site (i.e., next to a downed log or boulder).

     (2) Be sure that the location for the latrine would not be considered a good spot for a tentsite or kitchen by the next camper who uses the campsite.

   b. Decide on a shape

     (1) Square is the conventional shape.

     (2) Many prefer a rectangular trench.

     (3) Some find it easier to straddle a trench.

     (4) Rounding the corners of the latrine makes it easier to restore when closing it up.

   c. Cut out the sod and set it aside. Water the sod if necessary to maintain any vegetation growing in it.

   d. Dig the latrine 8 to 16 inches (20-40 cm.) deep, or down to the upper level of mineral soil. It is important to keep the latrine in the duff layer to help decompose the waste.

   e. Leave the soil next to the latrine along with a shovel or spade.

   f. Toilet paper

(1)   If used, it can either be left at the site or carried to the latrine by the user.

      (2)   Toilet paper that is left at the site runs the risk of getting wet from rain, even if it is bagged in plastic.

      (3)   Consider creative alternatives to toilet paper such as leaves, sticks, smooth rocks, etc.

  g.   To assure privacy while using the latrine, a marker such as a bandana can be tied around a nearby branch to indicate that it is occupied.

3. **Using the latrine**

  a.   Keep in mind good sanitary practices when using the latrine.

      (1)   Wash hands after use.

      (2)   Keep waste off the shovel.

      (3)   Keep waste in the latrine.

  b.   If toilet paper is used, burn it as completely as possible, being sure not to catch the nearby duff or litter on fire. Another alternative is to bag it for packing out or burning in a campfire.

  c.   Sprinkle just enough soil on the waste to keep flies and odor to a minimum – more than that will fill up the latrine too quickly.

  d.   Whether using a latrine, cathole, or outhouse, it is important that only human waste be put in them. Foreign matter may attract animals and also decompose too slowly. The following should **not** be disposed of with human waste:

      (1)   **Food waste** (See "Food Waste Disposal" lesson.)

      (2)   **Tampons or sanitary napkins**. These must be packed out for proper disposal. Adding 1-2 aspirin tablets with tampons or napkins in a double plastic bag will help keep odors to a minimum.

      (3)   **Trash**. Trash must either be completely burned or carried out.

4. **Closing the latrine**

  a.   Close the latrine when waste gets to within 3 or 4 inches (8-10 cm.) of the top.

  b.   Replace the soil.

  c.   Carefully replace the sod, trying to blend it in as naturally as possible.

d.   The LOD is responsible for closing latrines or delegating the responsibility. Either way, the LOD should check all latrine sites before leaving the campsite to be sure they have been closed properly.

C. **Catholes**

    1.   Catholes are small holes that are used once. They can be dug with a shovel. It is not a good idea to roll away a log or boulder to expose a hole, as entire communities of organisms inhabiting these areas are adversely affected.

    2.   They may be used by members of small groups in camp, or used during the day while traveling.

    3.   Catholes should not be used in heavily camped areas because of the increased chance of their discovery by others.

    4.   One way to minimize the amount of waste left in a camp latrine is to encourage the use of catholes while traveling during the day before getting into camp.

    5.   Like latrines, catholes should be located well away from trails and water sources.

    6.   After using a cathole, properly dispose of the toilet paper, cover the waste, and restore the site as naturally as possible.

D. **Urinating**

It is not essential to use a cathole or latrine to urinate. However, it is wise to use the same area near tentsites so group members know where people have urinated.

IV. **INSTRUCTIONAL STRATEGIES & MATERIALS:**

A. **Timing**

    1.   Although this lesson does not need to be taught until later in the course (within the first ten days), some initial instruction must be provided the first day.

B. **Strategies**

    1.   This is a good class for students to instruct. Although relatively simple, it requires good communication skills and the ability to give a demonstration.

    2.   Be sure to evaluate latrines on a daily basis and point out the good and bad points of each one.

3. Depending on the course location, special environmental considerations for depositing human waste should be mentioned. *Soft Paths* (see "Bibliography") is an excellent reference for sanitation in special environments such as deserts, rivers, lakes, coasts, alpine and arctic tundra, and snow and ice.

C. **Activities**
Encourage creativity by awarding the most creative "latrine-of-the-week." Make sure that the latrine meets all of the criteria for a good latrine, as well as being creative.

D. **Materials**
1. Shovel
2. Toilet paper and matches

12. Leadership

I. **GOAL**: To provide participants with a background of leadership theory and its components in order to reinforce field knowledge and practice.

II. **OBJECTIVES**:
   A. Participants will be able to define leadership both generically and in relation to wilderness education.
   B. Participants will understand and be able to list leadership styles.
   C. Participants will be able to understand and identify leadership cornerstones and traits.
   D. Participants will be able to explain the roles that personality and personal qualities play in leadership.
   E. Participants will be able to explain and understand the role followership plays in the leadership process.
   F. Participants will be able to explain and understand the importance of knowing one's strengths and limitations.
   G. Participants will be able to explain and understand the role communication plays in being a leader.
   H. Participants will be able to explain and understand the role of the leader and the importance of having one.
   I. Participants will be able to recognize and identify leadership styles in others as well as in themselves.

III. **CONTENT**:
   A. **Defining Leadership**
      1. "Leadership is a process which assists an individual or a group to identify goals and objectives and to achieve them. The leadership process is further defined by the need for some specific action, decision, or initiative by one or more persons acting in the leadership role. Outdoor Leadership means that the setting and program focus are directly

related to the natural or cultural environment" (Buell, 1983, p. 6).
2. "Any action that focuses resources toward a beneficial end" (Rosenbach & Taylor, 1984, p. xv).
3. "...the ability to plan and conduct safe, enjoyable expeditions while conserving the environment" (Petzoldt, 1984, p. 42).

B. **Leadership Styles**
The key components of leadership are mastering various leadership styles and developing the ability to adapt them to various situations. It is important to recognize one's leadership style patterns and that different leadership situations require different leadership styles. *Give examples.*
1. **The leadership continuum**
Leadership styles fit on a continuum. (See Figure 12-1.) At one end of the continuum, the leader makes the decision and tells the group what to do. At the other end, the group makes the decision and takes total responsibility for it.

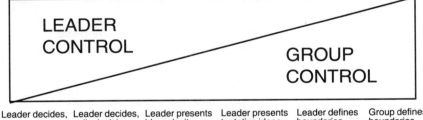

| Leader decides, announces decision | Leader decides, sells decisions | Leader presents ideas, invites questions | Leader presents tentative ideas subject to change | Leader defines boundaries, group decides | Group defines boundaries and decides |

Reprinted by permission from the publisher, Harvard Business Review

Figure 12-1 Leadership Style Continuum

2. **Primary leadership styles**
Historically, this continuum has been broken down into the following three primary leadership styles:
a. **Autocratic**
(1) The decision-making function resides primarily with the assigned leader (Buell, 1983).

(2)   Characteristics
         (a) Fast
         (b) Discourages a group commitment
         (c) Does not promote spontaneity or creativity within the group

      (3)   This is an effective method when the assigned leader has the most knowledge and experience. It is also effective in a dangerous situation when quick, decisive action must be taken. It is probably the most efficient style in terms of time and communication. *Give examples.*

b. **Democratic**

      (1)   The decision-making function resides with the group (Buell, 1983).

      (2)   Characteristics
         (a) Slow
         (b) Encourages a group commitment to the outcome
         (c) Produces greater initiative
         (d) May produce a disenchanted minority

      (3)   This style may be appropriate when the objective is to build group cohesiveness or when time is available. The democratic style is an important one to use when it is desirable to have a shared commitment or have the group accept responsibility for decisions. *Give examples.*

      (4)   While a democratic style may imply a group "vote," consensus is often used more effectively and is the ultimate expression of democracy. Consensus implies unanimity — that the whole group has agreed with the decision. Although it is often difficult and time-consuming to reach, consensus eliminates the disenfranchised minority of a democracy and maximizes group commitment.

c. **Laissez-faire**

      (1)   The decision-making function resides with the individual (Buell, 1983).

(2) This style should not be confused with consensus decision-making. Consensus assumes unanimity, while laissez-faire permits each individual to go his or her own way, independent of others within the group.

(3) Characteristics

  (a) Inhibits a sense of common group purpose

  (b) Inhibits the development of group cohesion

  (c) Allows for maximum individual freedom

(4) In wilderness education, an adaptation of this style may be used by instructors to empower a member of the group or the group as a whole, with the decision-making prerogative.

C. **Situational Leadership** (Hersey & Blanchard, 1982)

  1. Situational Leadership™ (see Figure 12-2) is based on three things:

    a. **The amount of direction (task behavior)**: The degree of specific guidance and instruction the leader must give the group to solve a problem.

    b. **The amount of socio-emotional support (relationship behavior)**: The degree of encouragement and instruction in helping the group work together effectively to accomplish its task.

    c. **The level of "maturity" of the group members**: The ability and readiness of individuals or a group to take responsibility for directing their own behavior.

  2. This model allows the leader to assess the group's readiness to accept responsibility for directing its own behavior, as well as monitor its progress through the stages of group development.

  3. Situational Leadership reinforces the fact that there is no "best" style of leadership and provides four styles:

    a. **Telling**: leader-centered. The leader "tells" the group what to do.

    b. **Selling**: problem-oriented vs. people-oriented leadership. The leader proposes solutions to problems.

c. **Participating**: shared decision making. The leader has the group actively involved in identifying and solving problems.

    d. **Delegating**: the leader delegates decision making and assumes a supportive role.

  4. The Situational Leadership styles parallel Jones' group development theory. (See the "Group Development" lesson for more detail.)

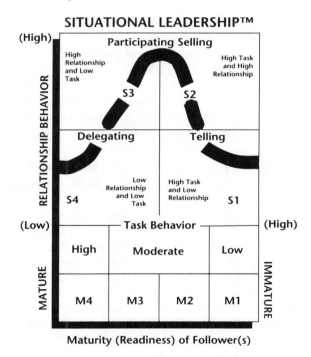

Paul Hersey/Ken Blanchard, MANAGEMENT OF ORGANIZATIONAL BEHAVIOR: Utilizing Human Resources, 4e, ©1982,p.152. Reprinted by permission of Prentice Hall, Englewood Cliffs, New Jersey.

Figure 12-2 Situational Leadership

D. **The Cornerstones of Leadership**

  1. **Definition and characteristics**

    a. The cornerstones of leadership are the critical components which determine and influence an individual's ability to lead. They are the building blocks which anchor the foundation upon which leadership is built.

b.   These cornerstones do not stand alone. They are connected by and work in harmony with leadership qualities and traits which together form a solid and balanced foundation for further leadership development.

    c.   Weakness in one area does not necessarily mean the structure is unsound. Just as a builder recognizes strengths and weaknesses that may exist in a building, so too must leaders acknowledge their own strengths and weaknesses.

2. **The four cornerstones**

    a.   **Intellectual potential**

       (1)   The ability to recognize, analyze, and synthesize information, thereby combining the creative thought processes of the right brain with the rational thought processes of the left brain.

       (2)   While intellectual potential alone does not make a leader (we all know intellectuals who would make terrible leaders), it is still a factor which determines a leader's capabilities.

    b.   **Personality**

       (1)   The distinctive emotional, behavioral, and temperamental traits which make up an individual.

       (2)   These qualities are considered a part of the individual's personality. While they can be developed and modified, they are a part of the individual's make-up regardless of whether or not they are in a leadership position.

       (3)   A characteristic of a dedicated leader is the extent to which that individual works on strengthening desirable personality characteristics (e.g., an individual has little patience but realizes this, and works on improving that characteristic in order to be a more effective leader).

    c.   **Knowledge**

       The cognitive component of leadership. It can be learned any number of ways:

(1) **Theoretical**
      (a) Reading
      (b) Observation
      (c) Listening
      (d) One of the limitations of theoretical knowledge is that, without experience, it provides too small a base for decision making, thus forcing the leader to be extremely conservative if objectives of safety and environmental protection are to be met.

    (2) **Experiential** – knowledge through doing.
      (a) If used appropriately, this is an excellent means of reinforcing knowledge and refining the decision-making process.
      (b) This is limited by the fact that, unless experience is processed, it is worthless. In other words, we don't learn from our mistakes unless we make a conscious effort to do so.

4. **Psychomotor skills**
This refers to the physical ability to do things, often among the most enjoyable parts of outdoor ventures. Although not the most critical component of outdoor leadership, psychomotor skills are necessary to:
    a. Provide for the safety of the group
    b. Pass on knowledge
    c. Provide a positive role model

E. **Leadership Qualities and Traits**
These are the attributes a leader should have. They can be broken down into three general groups: essential leadership qualities, leadership traits, and personal qualities.
1. **Essential leadership qualities:** Those qualities which are critical to effective leadership.
    a. **Quality decision-making ability**
      (1) Probably the most critical factor in leadership is the ability to make and/or facilitate quality decisions (i.e., decisions which are appropriate for the situation). See the

"Decision Making" lesson for a detailed discussion of the decision-making process.

 (2) Leaders with good decision-making abilities and a knowledge of their own limitations will be less likely to run into trouble.

 b. **Knowledge of one's strengths and limitations**

  (1) "Know what you know and know what you don't know."

  (2) This requires that leaders constantly self-assess themselves in order to evaluate their own strengths and weaknesses. Unless leaders can stay within their own limitations, they will not be truly safe leaders.

  (3) Leaders must be realists and not bluff either themselves or their clients.

 c. **Selflessness**

  To be effective in achieving group objectives, it is essential that leaders have the ability to put group needs above their own interests.

2. **Leadership traits:** Those qualities which are generally recognized as desirable in a leader.

 a. Achieves objectives

 b. Understands participants' needs

 c. Gets along with participants

 d. Is resourceful

 e. Gains confidence of participants

 f. Has the ability to analyze problems

 g. Is adaptable to situations

 h. Has the ability to arouse and develop interest

 i. Leads without dominating

 j. Has the ability to handle disciplinary problems

 k. Has the ability to inspire others

 l. Has the ability to lead informally

 m. Encourages participant leadership

 n. Has the ability to plan and organize

 o. Observes rules and regulations

 p. Takes proper care of equipment and property

 q. Uses time effectively

 r. Is safety conscious, but permits freedom of adventure

 s. Has the ability to serve as a role model

3. **Personal qualities**: The distinctive traits which make up the individual (Buell, 1983).
   a. Poise
   b. Cooperative attitude
   c. Self-discipline
   d. Tolerance
   e. Patience
   f. Concern for others
   g. Appearance
   h. Physical fitness
   i. Dependability
   j. Willingness to learn
   k. Effective speech
   l. Integrity
   m. Promptness
   n. Self-confidence
   o. Enthusiasm
   p. Initiative

F. **Leadership Execution**
   1. **The role and importance of the leader**
      a. Quite often the leader is thought of as the individual who handles emergencies. While this ability is of the utmost importance, it is the exceptional responsibility. The definitions of leadership imply a much broader role.
      b. The leader is not the person at the front of the line, but rather the person floating among the group, checking that everything is all right.
      c. The leader is an organizer who anticipates and tries to make things go smoothly, becoming a problem-solver as the need arises.
      d. Although contrary to the WEA philosophy, there are trips that operate on a leaderless philosophy. Without one individual taking overall responsibility for the group, the potential for problems greatly increases. As President Harry Truman said, "The buck stops here."
   2. **Communication**
      a. A leader will rarely get into trouble by overcommunicating, but may often get into trouble by undercommunicating.
      b. There is a tendency to overestimate the group's understanding of situations.

c. Leaders should take the time to explain as much as possible in every given situation. For example, if the group is taking a break, the leader should let everyone know how long it will be. Or, if unforeseen circumstances change the objectives of the trip, the leader should communicate those changes.

d. Communicating minimizes misunderstanding and lessens individual and group frustration.

3. **The leader as a role model**

a. A leader must serve as a role model and must not follow the creed, "Do as I say, not as I do."

b. Double standards must be minimized. If they must exist at all, the reason should be communicated and explained to the group.

c. The leader who serves as a good role model will develop a group of excellent followers.

4. **Followership**

a. **Definition**
"The American Camping Association defines followership as the ability to serve in a democratic group situation under leadership of a member of that group but still retain the capacity to suggest, criticize and evaluate, as well as serve in the project" (Buell, 1983, p. 8). Buell also lists additional qualities for being a follower:

(1) Stress the importance of the individual

(2) Accept a lesser role so the group can reach its goals

(3) Keep communication open with leaders and other followers

b. Good followership is as important as good leadership. Individuals should be committed to followership because:

(1) Without followers, goals will not be met.

(2) Being a good follower allows a leader to develop empathy for followership.

(3) Most people go through life primarily as followers. Unfortunately, just as leaders are not formally trained, neither are followers.

5. **Leading vs. instructing**
   Does a good leader have to be a good teacher? Does a good teacher have to be a good leader? It is generally recognized that a good teacher does not have to be a good leader, but a good leader must be a good teacher. Many feel good leaders are even better teachers.

6. **Recognizing and identifying leadership styles**
   An important means of developing positive leadership abilities is to recognize and identify the leadership styles of others. This can be done through observation and debriefings.

IV. **INSTRUCTIONAL STRATEGIES & MATERIALS:**
   A. **Timing**
   1. This lesson should be taught after participants have a good understanding of the Leader of the Day (LOD) concept and a number of the participants have had an opportunity to serve as LOD.
   2. It is important to reinforce the information in the lesson with examples — ideally, examples from the trip itself.
   3. It may be appropriate to teach a lot of this information informally, on an individual basis, or during debriefings, but it is critical to have a formal class on leadership to ensure that all components are covered.

   B. **Strategies**
   For participants to develop their leadership abilities to the greatest extent possible, it is important to:
   1. Let the LOD's take as active a role as possible.
      a. Let them take charge with as little interference as possible.
      b. Let them make mistakes, then help them constructively and positively.
   2. Have the LOD and the group evaluate leadership roles in terms of successes and failures. Also, have the LOD and the group describe the leadership styles, cornerstones, traits, and personal qualities exhibited.
   3. Encourage future LOD's to build on the previous leaders' strengths and weaknesses.
   4. Give participants time to grow.
   5. Communicate to the participants what they can do to improve.

6. Be objective — don't let personal likes and dislikes interfere with evaluating someone's leadership.
7. Understand that in group discussions, the instructor's words carry more weight than do students.

C. **Activity**:
Leadership Traits Activity
This activity allows participants to evaluate themselves and their peers in a non-threatening way in order to see both positive and negative leadership qualities they have exhibited during the trip. The primary purpose of this activity is for participants to increase their leadership qualities and observation abilities.

1. Before the activity, make two lists of leadership traits and personal qualities that have been observed during the trip. Pick out at least one positive and one negative quality for each participant.
2. Divide the group in two and give each group a list of observed traits of the other group.
3. Split the groups up for a predetermined length of time (30-45 minutes) to do the next two tasks (#4 and #5).
4. Ask each group to match one of the traits with a member of the other group and give an example of when the group member exhibited the quality in a positive way.
5. Ask each group to review the traits on their list and to discuss which traits have been exhibited during the trip.
6. Bring the groups back together to discuss what positive traits they found in the other group and what negative traits were offered within their own group.
7. Wrap up the discussion with an emphasis on:
   a. The importance of observing leaders and working on improving ourselves.
   b. The importance of self-analysis.
   c. The fact that we all have both positive and negative traits.

13. Nutrition and Rations Planning

I.   **GOAL:** To have participants plan food rations for wilderness outings with an understanding of the nutritional requirements involved.

II. **OBJECTIVES:**
A.   Participants will understand the importance of food in wilderness travel.
B.   Participants will be able to list and explain the body's nutritional needs.
C.   Participants will be able to list considerations in food planning.
D.   Participants will be able to explain the WEA ration planning philosophy.
E.   Participants will be able to explain how the "Total Food Planning" process works.
F.   Participants will be able to explain the role computers can play in food planning.

III. **CONTENT:**
A.   **Food Plays Important Roles In:**
1.   **Staying healthy**
Keeping well-nourished plays an instrumental role in fighting illness and disease.
2.   **Building and repairing body tissue**
3.   **Attitude**
Without good nutrition, disposition and attitude deteriorate rapidly.
4.   **Energy**
Food provides the energy that allows us to take part in physical activities.
5.   **Mental alertness**
Thought processes and decision-making ability deteriorate without good nutrition.

© 1992
The Wilderness Education Association
P.O. Box 89
Saranac Lake, New York 12983
(518) 891-2915 ext. 254

B. **Specific Nutritional Needs**
   1. **Calories**
     a. A calorie is a unit of heat used to measure the energy value of food. It takes one calorie to raise one gram of water one degree centigrade.
     b. Individual daily caloric needs range from approximately 1800 per day for a sedentary individual to over 6500 for an expedition member in severe weather.
     c. In general, individual daily caloric needs for wilderness travelers range between:
       (1) 2800 and 4000 in summer.
       (2) 3800 and 6000 in winter.
   2. **Carbohydrates**
     a. Carbohydrates provide short term energy.
     b. They should make up approximately 60% of an individual's diet.
     c. Carbohydrates are found in starches and sugars such as:
       (1) Pastas (macaroni, noodles, spaghetti)
       (2) Rice
       (3) Potatoes
       (4) Drink mixes
       (5) Candy
       (6) Fruit
   3. **Fats**
     a. Fats provide long term energy.
     b. They should make up approximately 20 - 25% of an individual's diet.
     c. Fats are found in:
       (1) Cheese
       (2) Nuts
       (3) Vegetable oil
       (4) Meats
       (5) Margarine
   4. **Protein**
     a. The body uses protein to provide for the building of cells and tissue such as skin and muscles.
     b. It should make up approximately 15 - 20% of an individual's diet.
     c. Proteins are made up of 22 amino acids. Of these 22, all but eight are produced in our

bodies. The other eight must be obtained
through proteins in food.

d. Complete proteins vs. incomplete proteins

  (1) **Complete proteins**

These include all eight of the essential
amino acids that the body cannot produce.
Therefore, they provide a full complement
of protein. Examples include:

    (a) Meats (pepperoni)

    (b) Fish

    (c) Soy products (soy flour, soy nuts)

  (2) **Incomplete proteins**

These include some, but not all eight of the
essential amino acids. Therefore, they do
not provide a full complement of protein.
Examples of incomplete proteins include:

    (a) Cereals (oats, Cream of Wheat,
Wheatena)

    (b) Vegetables and fruit

    (c) Legumes (beans, peanuts, lentils)

  (3) Incomplete proteins can be made complete
by combining two or more foods (e.g.,
beans and vegetables) together in the same
meal. Although this usually happens
naturally, it is helpful to be aware of this to
insure that complete proteins are
consumed regularly.

5. **Vitamins and minerals**

If participants consume a variety of foods and the
recommended high number of calories, vitamin and
mineral intake is generally adequate. Supplemental
vitamins and minerals are usually unnecessary.

6. **Water**

Water is a critical nutritional element.

a. Water aids in digestion.

  (1) It keeps cells healthy

  (2) It regulates body temperature

  (3) It helps to carry wastes out of the body

b. Times when the body is more susceptible to
dehydration:

  (1) Strenuous activity (water is lost through
perspiration)

(2) Higher altitudes (water is lost through increased respiration in drier air)
(3) Cold weather (water is lost through respiration and perspiration)
c. A minimum of 2-4 quarts in summer, and 3-4 quarts in winter should be consumed each day to prevent dehydration.

C. **Food Planning Considerations**
Depending on the objectives and length of the trip, the following criteria should be considered:
1. **Energy content**
The number of calories supplied by a food item in relation to its bulk and weight.
2. **Nutritional balance**
3. **Bulk and weight**
4. **Spoilage**
The risk of food spoiling varies with the season and region.
5. **Expense and availability**
Is it available, and if so, can the group afford it?
6. **Ease of packaging and handling**
a. Can it be packaged environmentally (i.e., in plastic rather than cans which, if accidentally left behind, would be less likely to decompose or burn than plastic)?
b. How easily can it be handled without spilling, etc.?
7. **Variety**
a. The longer the trip, the more important this becomes as a morale booster. Few people want to eat the same thing day after day.
b. The more variety, the better the chance of appealing to everyone's food tastes.
8. **Preparation time**
Can it be prepared in a reasonable amount of time?
9. **Supplementary wild foods**
a. Are they available?
b. Can they be harvested legally?
c. Are participants knowledgeable enough to prevent accidental poisoning?

d.   Can they be harvested without impacting the environment (e.g., plants chosen will be naturally replenished within a reasonable time)?

D. **Ration Planning**

    1. **"Total Food Planning"**

       a. **Definition**

         This process is based on determining caloric needs and ensuring that the group has enough food to meet caloric needs while staying within weight and budget constraints.

       b. **Planning criteria**

         (1) **Caloric needs**

           During summer months, between 3200 and 3750 calories are planned per person per day, depending on activity level and weather.

         (2) **Weight needs**

           Approximately 2 pounds of food per person per day is required during summer months.

         (3) **Budget needs**

           Nutritious meals can be provided for between $2.50 and $4.50 per person per day.

       c. **Advantages of "Total Food Planning"**

         (1) A large variety of foods can be used, allowing for an endless variety of meals.

         (2) Cooking can be spontaneous and creative.

         (3) It eliminates the need to plan specific meals. Individuals can eat what they want, when they want and, in general, should have enough food for the trip.

         (4) By minimizing pre-mixed meals and cooking from scratch, financial savings can be realized.

    2. **How "Total Food Planning" works** (See sample of the "Master Food List" in the appendix at the end of this chapter.)

       a. **Calories**

         Multiply the number of people (P) going on the trip times the number of days (D) of the trip times the minimum number of calories (C) to be brought per person per day. This is the

minimum number of calories needed for the
trip (e.g., 12(P) X 33(D) X 3500(C) = 1,386,000.
See line 103 column D of the "Master Food List").

b. **Weight**
Multiply the number of people (P) going on the
trip times the number of days (D) of the trip times
the maximum number of pounds (P) to be brought
per person per day. This is the maximum
number of pounds of food to be brought on the
trip (e.g., 12(P) X 33(D) X 2(P) = 792. See line
103 column B of the "Master Food List").

c. **Cost**
Multiply the number of people (P) going on the
trip times the number of days (D) of the trip
times the maximum amount of money ($) to be
spent per person per day. This is the maximum
amount of money to be spent on food for the
trip (e.g., 12(P) X 33(D) X $3.25 = $1287. See line
103 column F on the "Master Food List").

d. **Working with the results**
Use these figures and the planning
considerations to develop a food list which
meets calorie, weight, and cost criteria.

E. **Computers and the Food Planning Process**
Spreadsheet software can be used to save time and
anguish, making food planning easier.

1. A shopping list can be created that meets minimum
caloric needs and maximum pound and cost
parameters. Once the data base is established, at the
press of a button the computer will do all the
computations and generate food lists.

2. A nutritional analysis of the food selected for the trip
can be done.

IV. **INSTRUCTIONAL STRATEGIES & MATERIALS:**
A. **Timing**

1. Depending on how the course is designed, this
lesson can be taught as part of the shakedown (i.e., a
short trip at the beginning of a WEA course
designed to provide an intense philosophical
orientation and skills preparation for the remaining
time in the field) or near the end of the course.

a.   On most WEA courses, students plan their own rations as part of the shakedown exercise. In this case, this lesson should be taught the first day.

       b.   Some WEA affiliates pre-plan food for a trip and get participants involved in food planning at a later point. In this case, this lesson becomes a lower priority and is taught later in the course, using the trip as an example.

B. **Activities**

Have participants develop a rations plan and use it during a trip. Keep good records of what is brought and what is returned so caloric consumption can be tracked. It is much easier and more practical for this exercise to be done by tent groups rather than individually. This requires cooperation and is more practical than having participants compile separate lists and then combine food with their tent partners.

C. **Materials**

"Master Food List" (See appendix).

Master Food List

1 Wilderness Recreation Leadership Program
2 North Country Community College
3 20 Winona Ave.
4 Saranac Lake, NY 12983

	A	B	C	D	E	F
5	A	B	C	D	E	F
6	Names: Sample	Total -	12	Total -	33	
7		People		Days		
8		---------	---------	---------	---------	---------
9		Pounds	Calories	Total	Cost	Total
10		Ordered	per Pound	Calories	per LB.	Cost
11		---------	---------	---------	---------	---------
12	Apples - dried	10	1102	10563	$1.52	$14.57
13	Apricots - dried	14	1081	15081	$1.59	$22.18
14	Bacon - pieces	0	2836	0	$1.99	$0.00
15	Baking Powder	3	585	1883	$0.80	$2.58
16	Bagels	0	1800	0	$1.24	$0.00
17	Beef Base	3	1082	3484	$2.32	$7.47
18	Bread	0	1102	0	$1.05	$0.00
19	Brownie Mix	8	1828	13732	$1.33	$9.99
20	Bulgar	3	1621	5219	$0.32	$1.03
21	Candy - hard	11	1751	18535	$1.76	$18.63
22	Cashews	0	2604	0	$2.09	$0.00
23	Cheese Cake mix	5	3500	18524	$2.23	$11.80
24	Cheese: Cheddar	23	1826	41152	$1.94	$43.72
25	Mozzarella	21	1270	27259	$1.72	$36.92
26	Muenster	41	1671	68144	$1.66	$67.70
27	Colby	33	1786	59417	$1.75	$58.22
28	Chicken Base	2	1117	2397	$2.32	$4.98
29	Chili Base	1	1450	1556	$2.55	$2.74
30	Chocolate Bars	0	1650	0	$3.38	$0.00
31	Cocoa w/milk	26	1628	41931	$1.99	$51.25

© 1992
The Wilderness Education Association
P.O. Box 89
Saranac Lake, New York 12983
(518) 891-2915 ext. 254

		A	B Pounds Ordered	C Calories per Pound	D Total Calories	E Cost per LB.	F Total Cost
32	Coconut		3	2468	7765	$0.93	$2.93
33	Corn Meal		0	1610	0	$0.21	$0.00
34	Crackers		0	1828	0	$2.35	$0.00
35	Cream of wheat		0	1658	0	$1.12	$0.00
36	Dates		6	1243	8004	$1.12	$7.21
37	Eggs - freeze dried		0	2697	0	$6.83	$0.00
	1lb=32 eggs						
38	Egg Noodles		9	1760	15110	$0.61	$5.24
39	Fruit Drink - Orange		52	1950	100449	$0.99	$51.00
40	Lemon		0	1950	0	$0.99	$0.00
41	Fruit		0	1950	0	$0.99	$0.00
42	Tang		0	1950	0	$1.65	$0.00
43	Flour Unbleached		50	1650	82500	$0.19	$9.50
44	Whole Wheat		20	1651	33020	$0.31	$6.20
45	Gingerbread mix		12	1928	22760	$1.47	$17.35
46	Granola		0	2211	0	$1.30	$0.00
47	Ham - Cooked		0	1800	0	$3.00	$0.00
48	Honey		18	1379	25158	$0.78	$14.23
49	Hot Cereal (Wheatena)		5	1618	8682	$0.96	$5.15
50	Jello		4	1683	7225	$1.84	$7.90
51	Macaroni		18	1674	30540	$0.61	$11.13
52	Margarine		40	3387	134489	$0.57	$22.63
53	M & M's		9	2100	18029	$2.39	$20.52
54	Mighty Mush		5	1750	9390	$0.80	$4.29
55	Milk - powdered		23	1650	37950	$1.47	$33.81
56	Mushroom soup base		2	2000	4293	$3.44	$7.38
57	Nuts - mixed		3	2694	8673	$2.49	$8.02
58	Oatmeal		29	1672	48447	$0.29	$8.40
59	Onions - dried		3	1465	4717	$2.32	$7.47
60	Pancake Mix		19	1615	31197	$0.70	$13.52
61	Pancake syrup		4	1600	6868	$0.79	$3.39
62	Peanut Butter		20	2682	54687	$1.04	$21.21
63	Peanuts		14	2558	35687	$1.17	$16.32
64	Pepperoni		13	2255	29040	$4.40	$56.66
65	Peppers - dried		1	1000	1073	$17.80	$19.10
66	Popcorn		2	1642	3524	$0.27	$0.58
67	Potatoes - Sliced		4	1624	6971	$2.56	$10.99
68	Powder		3	1650	5312	$1.15	$3.70

	A	B	C	D	E	F
		Pounds Ordered	Calories per Pound	Total Calories	Cost per LB.	Total Cost
69	Prunes	6	1018	6555	$0.87	$5.60
70	Pudding - chocolate	3	1637	5270	$2.05	$6.60
71	vanilla	2	1637	3514	$2.05	$4.40
72	Raisins regular	25	1359	33544	$0.88	$21.72
73	golden	0	1368	0	$0.88	$0.00
74	Rice	12	1647	19443	$0.42	$4.96
75	Salami	00	2041	0	$4.40	$0.00
76	Salt	0	0	0	$0.16	$0.00
77	Sloppy Joe Base	1	1400	1502	$2.22	$2.38
78	Soup Blend w/ Dried Veggies	8	1600	12020	$5.60	$42.07
79	Sour Cream	2	1600	3434	$5.09	$10.92
80	Soy Nuts	8	1800	13522	$0.76	$5.71
81	Spaghetti	17	1674	28744	$0.61	$10.47
82	Sugar Brown	17	1700	29190	$0.70	$12.02
83	White	8	1700	12771	$0.36	$2.70
84	Sunflower seeds	9	2550	21893	$0.55	$4.72
85	Tea (Bags) reg - $/bag	0	0	0	$0.01	$0.00
86	spice - $/bag	0	0	0	$0.07	$0.00
87	Tomato Base	9	1350	11590	$6.58	$56.49
88	Trail mix	11	2000	21463	$1.74	$18.67
89	T V P Beef	4	1500	6439	$2.96	$12.71
90	Chicken	4	1500	6439	$2.96	$12.71
91	Ham	4	1500	6439	$2.96	$12.71
92	Vanilla	0	0	0	$14.16	$0.00
93	Vegetable Oil	13	4000	51512	$0.80	$10.30
94	Vinegar	0	54	0	$0.49	$0.00
95	Walnuts	5	2950	15829	$2.57	$13.79
96	Yeast	0	1250	0	$1.21	$0.00
97						
98	Total	Total 764		Total 1,421,396		Total $1,020.60
99	People -12					
100		Total		Total		
101	Total	Pounds		Calories		Total
102	Days - 33	Needed		Needed		Budget
103		Summer 792		Total 1,386,000		Total $1,287.00
104						

14. PackAdjustments

I. **GOAL**: To have participants fit and properly adjust their internal or external frame packs to an acceptable level of comfort while on the trail.

II. **OBJECTIVES**:
   A. Participants will be able to identify and describe the function of each of the major component parts of a pack's suspension system.
   B. Participants will be able to fit a pack to themselves and assist in properly fitting packs to others.
   C. Participants will be able to adjust their packs for stability and comfort while on the trail.

III. **CONTENT**:
   A. **Components of a backpack suspension system**
      1. **The external frame pack**
         a. **The frame**
            (1) **Description**
                Usually made of welded tubular aluminum, although occasionally made of "high tech" plastics.
            (2) **Purpose**
                (a) It is designed to hold a heavy load with sufficient stability and rigidity, allowing the packer to walk in safety and comfort.
                (b) The rigidity of the frame allows the weight of the load to be distributed evenly to the body of the packer through the suspension system.

© 1992
The Wilderness Education Association
P.O. Box 89
Saranac Lake, New York 12983
(518) 891-2915 ext. 254

b. **Waist belt**
   (1) **Description**
      (a) A heavily padded, and usually contoured, wrap-around belt located at the bottom of the pack frame.
      (b) The belt is usually attached to the frame with nylon webbing straps, clevis pins, or cinch belts.
      (c) The waist belt usually comes in various sizes (e.g., small, medium, or large) and is usually equipped with an adjustable length of nylon webbing which can accommodate a variety of waist sizes.
      (d) The waist belt has a quick-release buckle of hardened plastic or metal.
   (2) **Purpose**
      This belt fits snugly around the waist of the packer so that the padded portion of the belt rests squarely on the hips. This transfers the weight of the load to the pelvic girdle and onto the thighs of the packer. The pelvis and legs are the strongest parts of the body and best designed to carry weight.

c. **Waist belt stabilizers**
   (1) **Description**
      If included on the pack, these are located on the outer circumference of the waist belt near each of the hips.
   (2) **Purpose**
      (a) These short lengths of nylon webbing and buckles connect the rear of the waist belt directly to the bottom of the pack frame.
      (b) When tightened, these two stabilizers pull the pack frame toward the packer's hips, creating a more snug fit while walking.

d. **Shoulder pads**
   (1) **Description**
      These heavily-cushioned nylon pads are attached to a cross bar on the upper third

of the pack frame and to the base of the pack frame by adjustable webbing straps.

  (2) **Purpose**

    (a) When properly fitted over the packer's shoulders, these pads assist in carrying some of the pack's weight.

    (b) More importantly, they help stabilize the pack by drawing the frame and load close to the back so that most of the weight will ride directly on the pelvis.

e. **Shoulder pad stabilizers**

  (1) **Description**

These nylon webbing and buckle assemblies connect each of the shoulder pads to a cross bar on the upper third of the pack. When these straps are pulled tight, the pack frame is brought snug against the upper back and shoulder area of the packer.

  (2) **Purpose**

When tightened, these straps help minimize some of the rocking and swaying of the pack frame when walking.

f. **Mesh back band**

  (1) **Description**

This wide nylon mesh band is drawn tightly across the two vertical legs of the external frame.

  (2) **Purpose**

    (a) When properly taut, this back band presses against the shoulder blades and prevents the packer's back from coming in contact with any of the metal tubing of the pack frame.

    (b) On some packs, this band creates enough space to allow for some air circulation between the pack and the person wearing the pack.

g. **Cross-chest sternum strap**

  (1) **Description**

This nylon webbing with a quick-release buckle is attached to the front and middle of each of the shoulder pads.

    (2) **Purpose**

        (a) When this strap is drawn across the chest and pulled tight, the two shoulder pads are pulled toward the packer's sternum.

        (b) This keeps the shoulder pads securely in place, increases comfort, and helps reduce some of the side to side rocking motion common to many external frame packs.

2. **The internal frame pack**

  a. **The frame**

    (1) **Description**

        (a) As the name suggests, the frame of the internal frame pack is not visible because it is contained inside the pack itself.

        (b) Depending on the specific design of the pack, the metal staves that give the pack its rigidity are usually located in concealed pouches within the wall of the pack bag which is closest to the packer's back.

    (2) **Purpose**

        (a) An internal frame pack is more flexible, rides closer to the body, and is more responsive to the packer's subtle turns and shifts than an external frame pack.

        (b) The absence of a frame makes this pack preferable in heavy brush where it is less likely to catch or snag on branches.

  b. **The suspension system**

    Description

    (1) Most internal frame packs have suspension systems made up of basically the same components as those of better external frame packs (i.e., waist belt, waist belt stabilizers, shoulder pads, etc.).

    (2) Internal frame packs usually have fairly sophisticated adjustments for properly fitting the torso length of the packer. Each

111

model's apparatus must be understood and adjusted to ensure a proper fit.

(3) For a proper fit, the staves should be removed from their pouches, bent to conform to the curves of the packer's back, and then returned to their pouches.

(4) Trace a line from the top of the pelvis around to the spine. The bottom of the stave should be approximately 4 inches below this line when measured against the packer's spine.

B. **Fitting the Pack**
    Ideally, packs should contain at least 30-35 pounds (14-16 kg.) of equally distributed weight when being fitted to the packer.

1. **Fitting the waist**

    a. Loosen the waist belt stabilizers so that the waist belt is free to wrap around the waist and conform to the packer's body.

    b. Adjust the waist buckle so that when joined, it is located just below the belly button.

    c. Suck in the stomach and pull the waist belt tight. The top of the waist belt should be about 1" above the pelvic crest.

    d. Pull the waist belt stabilizers tight. The bottom section of the pack should feel comfortably secure against the hips.

2. **Fitting the torso**

    a. The pack suspension system and frame must fit properly between the base of the neck and the shelf that is formed by the small of the back and buttocks. This distance between the shoulders and the lower back is known as torso length.

    b. After fitting the waist belt to the hips, check the nylon mesh back band of the pack.

        (1) The middle of the back band should pass squarely across the points of both shoulder blades. This should keep the packer's back off the frame of an external frame pack or maximize comfort of an internal frame pack.

        (2) Adjust if necessary.

c. Tighten the shoulder pads.
    (1) The top portion of the shoulder pads should curve slightly over the shoulder of the packer and then attach to the pack.
    (2) For a proper fit, the load stabilizer should attach to the shoulder pad between the collar bone and the ridge of muscle along the top of the shoulder. (See Figure 14-1).
    (3) If the shoulder pad/load stabilizer is not fitted properly, adjust the shoulder harness where it attaches to the pack, either up or down, until it fits as described above.

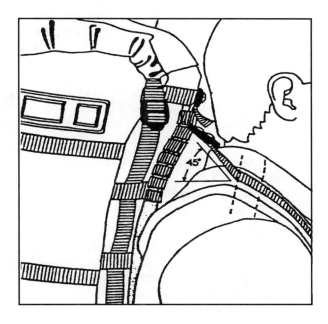

Reprinted by permission from Madden, Boulder, CO

Figure 14-1 Pack Adjustments

d. If fitted properly, the shoulders should feel as if they are stabilizing the movement of the load without accepting a great deal of the weight of the pack.

e. Once the shoulder pads conform to the torso length, check the shoulder pad stabilizer straps.
 (1) The stabilizer strap should angle up and away from the clavicle and attach to the pack at an angle of approximately 45° (see Figure 14-1).
 (2) When pulled tight, this strap should draw the top half of the pack load snug against the shoulders, thus placing the weight more directly over the hips.

C. **Adjusting the Pack on the Trail**
1. While walking, packers should constantly be adjusting the waist belt, the shoulder pads, and the stabilizers to improve the level of comfort.
2. Should the hips get tired or sore, loosen the waist belt to allow the shoulders to carry more of the weight.
3. Should the shoulders become sore, tighten the waist belt and loosen the shoulder pads so that all weight is transferred to the pelvis. By alternating the loosening of each shoulder strap, one shoulder can rest and then the other.

IV. **INSTRUCTIONAL STRATEGIES & MATERIALS:**
 A. **Timing**
 This class is usually conducted very early in the backpacking portion of the course.

 B. **Strategies**
 1. The sections about components (A.) and pack fitting (B.) can be taught as a lecture/demonstration and be incorporated into the "Pack Packing" lesson.
 2. Pack adjustments are usually taught using teachable moments on the trail as problems naturally arise.
 3. Rest stops are a particularly good time to introduce pack adjustment terminology and make suggestions for fine tuning a pack for proper fit.

 C. **Materials**
 1. External frame pack
 2. A packed internal frame pack

15. Pack Packing

I. **GOAL:** To have participants pack a neat, well-balanced, and systematically organized backpack which is comfortable to wear and efficient to use while traveling in the backcountry.

II. **OBJECTIVES:**
   A. Participants will understand and be able to describe the major considerations in packing a pack for wilderness travel.
   B. Participants will demonstrate an ability to pack items for accessibility on the trail.
   C. Participants will demonstrate an ability to pack a well-balanced pack that is safe for travel over a variety of different terrains.
   D. Participants will understand and be able to explain the reasons for distributing weight in the pack.
   E. Participants will develop a system of pack organization which allows for efficient packing and inventory of gear.

III. **CONTENT:**
   C.B.S. = Conveniently Balanced System
   This abbreviation can be used to remind participants of the basic considerations in efficient backpacking.
   A. **Convenience**
      A pack which is organized so that it permits access to its most-needed contents greatly enhances the packer's efficient use of time and energy.
      1. The itinerary for the day should be considered when organizing the pack.
         a. Arrangement of equipment on and in the pack should reflect the probability of that equipment's use during the day.
         b. External pack pockets should hold items that will be used most frequently during the day.

© 1992
The Wilderness Education Association
P.O. Box 89
Saranac Lake, New York 12983
(518) 891-2915 ext. 254

Such items include water bottle, matches, toilet paper, trail snacks, foot care kit, sunglasses, bug repellent, camera, etc.

c. Other equipment that will be used for traveling or weather changes should also be securely strapped, lashed, or pocketed on the outside of the pack. Such items might include a pack raincover, ice axe, climbing rope, crampons, etc.

2. Equipment that may be needed in an emergency should be easily accessible. Such items might include first aid kit, repair kit, water purification system, rain fly, etc.

   a. The location of these items should be known to all members of the group.

   b. Keys to the emergency evacuation vehicle should be packed in a safe location that is known to all, or hidden at the vehicle.

   c. In cold or wet weather, rain gear and extra insulating clothing should be packed near the top of the pack or in a sheltered external pocket so that they can be reached during rest breaks.

3. Items not usually needed until arrival at the campsite should be packed inside the pack bag. Such items might include extra clothes, stove, pots and pans, food bags, flashlight, personal toilet kit, tent, etc.

4. Items of gear requiring special protection should be packed inside waterproof or water repellent stuffsacks.

   a. Extra clothing should be stuffed into waterproof, coated nylon or plastic sacks and packed near the bottom of the pack.

   b. Cameras and eyeglasses should be packed in cases and stored in the pack when not in use.

   c. Sleeping bags and sleeping pads should be stuffed inside a waterproof sack and packed in the bottom of the pack.

B. **Balance**

A well-balanced pack with properly distributed weight adds to the safety and comfort of the packer.

1. **Weight distribution and comfort**

   a. Heavy loads are most comfortably carried when the weight is placed directly in line with the largest and strongest bones and muscles of

the body (i.e., the pelvic girdle and upper thigh
bones and the muscles of the thighs and buttocks).

(1) The heaviest part of the pack should be
centered as close to the body and as near
to the top of the spinal column/base of the
neck area as possible. The load should be
centered between the shoulder blades.

(2) When packing the pack, the heaviest
single item of equipment (e.g., tent or
food) should be packed in or on the top
half of the pack and as close to the
packer's back as possible.

b. Heavy loads are most comfortably carried
when they are balanced left to right, top to
bottom, and front to back.

(1) **Balance left to right**
Items of similar weight should be packed
on opposite sides of the pack so that
neither side of the body is uncomfortably
overburdened. For example, if a fuel bottle
is packed in the upper left external pocket,
a water bottle can be packed in the upper
right external pocket.

(2) **Balance top to bottom**
Heavy weights near the top of the pack
should be counter-balanced by weight
near the bottom of the pack or frame. For
example, a tent that is lashed on the top of
an extended pack frame could be counter-
balanced by a sleeping bag and pad
attached to the bottom of the frame.

(a) Heavy items should not be placed so
high on the pack frame that they tip
the packer forward.

(b) Sleeping bag stuff sacks on the
bottom of the frame should not be so
overloaded that they pull the packer
backward.

(3) **Balance front to back**
Heavier items should be placed as close as
possible to the packer's back to minimize
pulling the packer backwards.

117

c.   With internal frame packs or daypacks that lack protective cushioning, an ensolite pad or sweater/jacket should be placed along the interior pack wall closest to the packer's back to protect from the edges of rigid equipment (e.g., pots, stoves, plastic food containers, etc.).

2. **Weight distribution and safety**

    a.   Terrain should influence the way that weight is distributed in the pack.

        (1) **Flat, easily-traveled terrain:** for maximum comfort, pack the heaviest weight high and close to the shoulders.

        (2) **Rough terrain, steep inclines, dead falls:** the pack weight should be distributed slightly lower toward the middle of the back, allowing for greater balance and mobility while twisting or turning.

        (3) **Boulder hopping, river crossing, traversing:** the weight of the pack should be very low on the back to lower the body's center of gravity and maximize balance. Some comfort may be sacrificed with the weight in this position.

    b.   Items that should be isolated from food and clothing, such as fuel bottles and stoves, should be packed in the outside pockets of the pack.

C. **System**

A pack that is organized with an efficient and consistent system speeds the process of daily packing and aids in maintaining an accurate inventory of equipment.

1. A personal "system" of pack organization allows the packer to load the pack easily, locate individual equipment quickly, and keep track of gear.

2. Some individual items can be grouped together and packed in separate stuff sacks.

    a.   **Toilet kit:** toothbrush, toothpaste, comb, hand cream, etc.

    b.   **Clothes bag:** socks, underwear, bandanas, etc.

    c.   **Food bag:** rations, bear rope, spice kit, etc.

    d.   **Personal repair kit:** pack parts, nylon cord, wire, small tools, etc.

    e.   **Ditty bag:** flashlight, extra batteries, shoelaces, cards, etc.

3. Packers should strive to keep their packs stream-lined and neat.

    a. All equipment should be placed either inside the pack bag, in pockets, or securely lashed to the pack frame. No odds and ends should protrude from the pack to catch on branches, poke other hikers, or wriggle free.

    b. Soft items like clothing should be stuffed between rigid equipment in the pack. This maximizes the efficient use of space and minimizes rattling, squeaking, or shifting of contents while walking.

    c. Sleeping bag stuff sacks and tents should be tightly and very securely lashed to the pack frame. Nylon webbing with appropriate buckles works well for this. A clove hitch is particularly useful for securing sleeping bag straps to the pack frame.

    d. Tent poles, ice axes, etc., should be lashed or strapped along the vertical line of the pack or horizontally so equipment does not extend beyond the width of the packer's body. If the packer can fit through a gap between trees or rock, the pack should follow easily.

    e. All extra lengths of pack cord, webbing, or stuff sack drawstrings should be doubled up, tied off, and tucked in so they do not hang loosely from the pack and catch on branches, etc.

4. Once a system has been developed that suits a packer's needs, it should be used consistently. Most items in the pack should be packed the same way and in the same place. An efficient system will even allow for small adjustments due to itinerary or terrain.

IV. **INSTRUCTIONAL STRATEGIES & MATERIALS:**
    A. **Timing**
    Pack packing is usually taught very early in the course, preferably before the first full day on the trail.

    B. **Strategies**
    1. This lesson may be taught as a lecture/demonstra-tion in which the instructors display all of their own gear, describe their own system, and pack their pack

while explaining the reasons for what they are doing. Immediately after the class, participants should pack their own gear.

2. A second method of teaching this lesson may be used with more experienced packers. After being on the trail for one or two days, have one or two group members lay out their gear and explain their ideas about packing. Participants may discuss the pros and cons of various approaches and arrive at many of the same understandings that would come through a more direct approach.

3. For younger participants, a discussion may be initiated by using a very poorly packed pack as the focus for a contest (e.g., "Find 10 things wrong with this pack"). Use the ensuing discussion to highlight the main points of packing theory.

4. Younger participants can also be taught by having them pack by "rooms" of the "house." For example, they can pack the "kitchen," which would include pots, pans, food, stove, utensils, etc.

5. Use teachable moments to point out positive and negative qualities of various packing strategies used by members of the group. With younger participants, a "Pack-of-the-Day" prize may be awarded to encourage the proper technique.

C. **Materials**
A backpack and all of its contents. If the group is using internal and external packs, it is best to demonstrate with both.

16. Personal Hygiene

by Mary Vance

I. **GOAL**: To have participants be aware of personal hygiene from both a social and safety perspective.

II. **OBJECTIVES**:
   A. Participants will be able to explain the part that personal hygiene plays in the success of a backcountry trip.
   B. Participants will be able to understand and practice the techniques that prevent potential health or personal problems.

III. **CONTENT**:
   A. **Importance of Personal Hygiene**
      1. Personal cleanliness contributes to positive expedition behavior.
         a. It shows consideration for tentmates and other group members.
         b. It helps to raise spirits and contributes to a feeling of overall well-being.
      2. It contributes to the positive role model image that leaders should maintain.

   B. **Bathing and Washing**
      1. Bathe and wash clothes as regularly as possible. The proper techniques are covered in the "Bathing and Washing" lesson.
      2. Spot washing can be done when time or weather conditions are not conducive to bathing.
      3. Major areas for spot bathing include armpits, crotch, feet, hands, teeth, and hair.

© 1992
The Wilderness Education Association
P.O. Box 89
Saranac Lake, New York 12983
(518) 891-2915 ext. 254

C. **Safety and Health**
1. **Feet**
   It is very important to keep feet in good condition, as they are a major mode of transportation in the backcountry. Evacuations have occurred because foot care has been neglected.
   a. NO BARE FEET! Footwear should be worn when in camp and when circumstances dictate (e.g., stony, rocky, or otherwise unsafe beach areas).
       (1) Sticks, stones, glass, etc., can cut and puncture feet.
       (2) Dirt can easily enter open wounds.
   b. Keep feet as clean and dry as possible.
       (1) Wet, warm environments promote bacterial or fungal growth.
       (2) Irritants such as sand or dirt between toes will encourage blistering.
       (3) Wash and use powder when needed.
   c. Treat hot spots immediately. Keep blisters clean and covered. (See "Trail Techniques: Advanced".)
2. **Hands**
   a. Washing hands frequently is important, especially when cooking. Hands carry germs and bacteria which are easily transmitted to mouth and food.
   b. Hand cream helps prevent dry skin cracks which are painful and can become infected.
3. **Sunburn**
   a. The danger of sunburn is higher when on water or snow, or at higher altitudes.
   b. Areas most susceptible are face, neck, shoulders, and eyes.
   c. Avoid potential problems by wearing sunscreen, ZnO_2, sunglasses, and a hat.

D. **Miscellaneous Considerations**
1. Dispose of used tampons by carrying them out in a zippered plastic bag or by burning them in a very hot fire.
2. Avoid sharing eating utensils.

3. Sterilize utensils by immersing them in boiling water for about 30 seconds before using.
4. Clean water bottles regularly, especially the screw threads in the lid. This and occasional sterilization will keep mold from growing and kill harmful bacteria.

IV. INSTRUCTIONAL STRATEGIES & MATERIALS:

A. **Timing**

This class is best taught early in the trip to set a tone of personal cleanliness and safety.

B. **Strategies**

1. A skit can be useful to introduce the subject matter.
2. In grizzly bear country or country where black bears present a potential problem:
    a. Using scented lotion, soaps, or deodorants may attract the attention of bears or mask human scents.
    b. Wash early in the day so that residual smells will dissipate before night.

17. Stove Operation

I. **GOAL**: To have participants properly operate a backpacking stove and know when it is appropriate to utilize a stove versus a fire.

II. **OBJECTIVES**:
   A. Participants will be able to start and operate one type of backpacking stove.
   B. Participants will know and be able to practice safety considerations in stove use.
   C. Participants will know proper stove terminology.
   D. Participants will know the considerations in handling and using stove fuel.
   E. Participants will understand environmental considerations in stove use.
   F. Participants will be able to care for the stove and deal with minor stove idiosyncrasies.
   G. Participants will be able to properly pack the stove for transport.

III. **CONTENT**:
   A. **Environmental Considerations**
      Use a stove when:
      1. Firewood is scarce (i.e., dead and down firewood cannot be readily found).
      2. The area is heavily camped.
      3. There is concern that the firewood supply will not readily replenish itself.
      4. There is any doubt about what the environmental impact might be.

   B. **General Stove Safety**
      1. Reinforce the idea that using the stove is probably the second most dangerous thing done on the course. (The first, most likely, is traveling in vehicles.)

2. As long as some basic safety considerations are followed, there shouldn't be any problems.
3. Considerations for stove location:
   a. Level area
   b. Stable area
   c. Non-flammable surroundings
   d. Protection from the wind
   e. Not in a tent unless there are no other options
      (1) If you must cook in a tent, do not start the stove in the tent.
      (2) Be sure there is adequate ventilation, since CO_2 fumes can be toxic in the close quarters of a tent.
      (3) Check with the agency sponsoring the group, since policies vary regarding stoves in tents (e.g., cooking in tents is not permitted in Boy Scouts of America policy).
      (4) Cooking in tents should be considered a last resort, winter-time activity.
4. If the stove should flare up and/or burst into flames:
   a. If possible, turn the stove off.
   b. Smother the stove with a billy can or other appropriate object.
   c. Do not use water to extinguish the flame. This will only help spread the fire. Fuel is lighter than water and will stay on top of it.

C. **Filling the Stove**
   1. **Safety considerations**
      Judgment dictates the following considerations:
      a. No open flame should be nearby (i.e., other lit stoves, candles, cigarettes, etc.).
      b. Fill the stove in a different location than where it will be lit and used. Any fuel that may have been spilled when the stove was filled could ignite when the stove is operating.
      c. The stove should be cool before filling.
   2. **The fuel bottle**
      a. Be careful not to lose any washers to the fuel bottle cap. The fuel bottle will leak without them.
      b. Be careful not to cross-thread the fuel bottle cap threads.

3. **The stove**
   a. Be careful not to lose the stove fuel tank cap. Place it where you can easily find it.
   b. Follow the manufacturer's directions to determine how much to fill the stove. Most stoves should be filled three-quarters full. Overfilling a stove does not allow enough space for the fuel to vaporize, creating a hazard in which pure fuel could ignite rather than fuel vapors.
   c. Once the stove has been filled, replace the stove tank fuel cap and the fuel bottle cap securely.
   d. It is expedient to fill the stove before each use.
      (1) The fuel won't run out in the middle of cooking a meal.
      (2) The stove can be filled without having to wait for it to cool.

D. **Stove Terminology**
   Explain all the parts of the stove and their functions.

E. **Stove Operation**
   1. **Stove starting**
      a. Explain and demonstrate how to start the stove using the manufacturer's operating instructions.
         (1) Light the match before turning on the gas
         (2) Hold the match upside down so it will burn better.
      b. *Explain the principles of how the specific stove being used for the course operates.*
      c. If using a stove on snow, some insulation (e.g., a small ensolite pad) can be placed below it to prevent it from sinking into the snow.
   2. **Once the stove has warmed up**
      a. Save fuel by having food ready to heat.
      b. Use gloves.
         (1) Minimize the chance of getting burned.
         (2) They can be used as pot holders.
   3. **Turning the stove off**

F. **Packing the Stove**
   1. Let the stove cool before packing it.
   2. Be sure it is protected so it won't get damaged or damage other items in the pack.

3. Release fuel pressure by loosening the cap but be sure to retighten it securely, making sure the on/off valve is in the "off" position.
4. Pack the stove upright to minimize the chance of fuel leakage.
5. Pack the stove well away from food items to prevent potential contamination.

IV. INSTRUCTIONAL STRATEGIES & MATERIALS:

A. Timing

1. This is usually taught the first morning before breakfast. Participants are told to bring the stoves and fuel bottles to class so they can go over the parts as the instructor does. After the class, participants can start their stoves and cook breakfast while instructors help out as needed.
2. This class is usually taught in conjunction with the first cooking class so participants can immediately put their knowledge into practice.
3. Stove maintenance is taught using teachable moments or later in the course.

B. Activities

Initiate a discussion of the advantages and disadvantages of stoves vs. fires.

C. Materials

1. Stove
2. Stove operating instructions
3. Fuel bottle with fuel
4. Matches
5. Stove storage container (stuff sack, etc.)
6. Stove repair kit

18. Teaching Technique

I.   **GOAL**: To have participants develop a basic competency as effective teachers in the field.

II. **OBJECTIVES**:
    A.   Participants will be able to describe and practice the basic skills needed for teaching informally while in the field.
    B.   Participants will recognize and effectively use opportunities for "teachable moments."
    C.   Participants will be able to discuss the major considerations in preparing a formal class in the field.
    D.   Participants will be able to discuss the advantages and disadvantages of various methodologies which can be employed in a formal class in the field.
    E.   Participants will demonstrate a minimum competency in the necessary skills for teaching in the field.

III. **CONTENT**:
    A. **Reflections on Teaching**
        1. **Teaching as a sharing of power**
            a.   Knowledge is power. Knowledge enables students to exercise influence and control over self, others, and the environment.
            b.   When teachers use and share their knowledge, they should recognize and responsibly exercise the power that they wield. Teachers must understand the potential they have for effecting life-changing decisions in their students.
        2. **Teaching as creative expression**
            a.   All teaching relies on effective interpersonal communication. There are as many means of communication as there are teachers.
            b.   There is no "best way" to teach. All teachers must find ways that are most effective for

© 1992
The Wilderness Education Association
P.O. Box 89
Saranac Lake, New York 12983
(518) 891-2915 ext. 254

themselves and their students within the
context of their own personalities, talents, and
teaching and learning styles.

 c. Teaching is an extremely personal endeavor. It
engages the individual's full repertoire of
intelligence, imagination, enthusiasm, judgment, and wit in creating and effectively
using educational experiences.

3. **Teaching as an act of caring**

 a. For learning to occur, the learner admits
ignorance, at least temporarily. Students trust
and presume that this ignorance or innocence
will not be unfairly exploited.

 b. The teacher should recognize the vulnerability
of students and genuinely care for their
physical and emotional well-being.

B. **Strategies in Teaching Outdoors**

1. **The "grasshopper" approach** (Petzoldt, 1984)

 a. Teaching in the backcountry involves learning
many things about a wide range of subjects in a
very short time.

 b. Since the safety and comfort of expedition
participants require that many subjects and
skills be taught quickly, it is common for
instructors to "hop" from one subject to
another as circumstances permit.

  (1) In this "grasshopper" approach, the
subject or skill is introduced,
demonstrated, and then applied in close
sequence, maximizing immediate
understanding and retention.

  (2) After initially introducing a subject or skill,
it can be approached at a later time and
further developed.

 c. Since the "grasshopper" approach allows the
sequence of subjects to remain flexible, classes
can be postponed until the most effective time
or environment for teaching them is
encountered.

2. The "teachable moment"
   a. Teachable moments are lessons presented spontaneously and inspired by specific situations or events encountered during the day.
   b. The use of "teachable moments" impels students to recognize that opportunities for learning occur constantly during a backcountry expedition. Students should be encouraged to recognize and identify these opportunities.
   c. **Teachable moments on the trail**
      (1) Once a teaching opportunity is recognized, concentrate on it intensely. Make sure the entire group recognizes the opportunity for learning and is not distracted by other concerns.
      (2) Ask students to describe the situation and its implications. This will help students to focus attention and retain pertinent details for later discussion.
      (3) Clarify the subject right away. Repeat whatever observations and conclusions the group may reach for all to hear. Relate the observations and conclusions to the broader objectives of the course.
      (4) Though errors in skills or judgment may provide excellent "teachable moments," be sure not to subject individuals to unnecessary embarrassment or ridicule. Try to depersonalize the situation so that expedition behavior and attitude is not adversely affected. Thank the expedition member for providing an opportunity to use them as a constructive example.
   d. **Informal "teachable moments"**
      (1) Many valuable insights can be "taught" through casual conversation or small group social discussion. When handled well, these dialogues can yield dramatic results in terms of a student's personal growth and understanding.
      (2) **Suggestions for handling informal "teachable moments"**

(a) Listen very attentively to student conversations and questions, anticipating the potential for helping identify or clarify important points.

(b) Evaluate the appropriateness of using specific conversations or discussions as teaching opportunities. Some feelings or questions are better left unexplored.

(c) Assuming the moment is appropriate, ask questions which will help identify a potentially significant opportunity. Questioning should provoke simple recognition of the facts and proceed to more complex thinking, such as analysis, synthesis, and evaluation.

(d) Be patient in reaching the desired outcome. Since students possess different levels of intellectual ability, they will reach their own conclusions in different ways and at different times. Conversations should allow students to explore ideas and their implications at their own pace.

(e) The teacher must be willing to look objectively at his or her own feelings so that students can freely express their own beliefs. The instructor may ultimately express personal views, being mindful to justify or support them, but only after students have had an opportunity to freely express themselves.

(f) If understandings are reached during the conversation, they should be clearly articulated in a summary statement so that everyone may grasp the concept(s).

3.   **Formal presentations**
   a.   **Organizational concerns**
     (1)   **Selecting a site**
       (a)   **Weather**
         Students should be sheltered from exposure to sun, wind, rain, or extremes of temperature.
       (b)   **Environmental impact**
         Select a natural amphitheater that is away from distracting influences and where the environmental damage from a large group will be minimized.
       (c)   **Safety**
         Select a safe site (both for participants and spectators).
       (d)   **Comfort**
         Students should be able to sit comfortably but attentively.
     (2)   **Timing of a class**
       (a)   Schedule classes in the morning when most people are fresh and alert.
       (b)   Announce class time well in advance so that camp chores are completed.
       (c)   Insist that students be on time and start classes promptly at the announced time.
       (d)   Allow for break time, stretching time, etc., during class to maintain student attention and comfort, and try to keep classes as short as possible.
     (3)   Make sure class teachers and student participants are fully informed of the subject or skills being taught before the class meets.
       (a)   All participants should know what materials (e.g., notebooks, equipment, etc.) will be needed for class.
       (b)   Teachers should be given adequate time to organize their lesson plans and teaching strategies.

b. **Communication skills**
 (1) **Speaking skills**
  (a) Speak clearly, loudly, and slowly so that all will understand.
  (b) Use a vocabulary that is appropriate for the subject and the group.
  (c) Establish eye contact with students and speak to them.
  (d) Use prepared notes as a reference, don't read from them.
  (e) Get the complete attention of the audience before proceeding with the class.
  (f) Vary the pitch and tone of the voice frequently for emphasis.
  (g) Use non-abrasive, courteous words. Refrain from slang or profanity unless specifically called for.
  (h) Refrain from using "inside" humor in front of the whole group. Such activity may exclude some members of the group from a sense of participation.
 (2) **Listening skills**
  (a) Listen attentively to student questions and responses, concentrating on the main points and specifics of each.
  (b) Listen courteously without interrupting unnecessarily and without distracting or mocking the questioner or speaker.
  (c) Listen patiently and allow students sufficient time to formulate questions or respond. Silence can be the sound of a mind working.
  (d) Listen empathetically and try to learn what is meant as well as what is said. Be aware of feelings and emotions, and encourage students who are reluctant to express themselves.
 (3) **Non-verbal communication**
  (a) Allow enthusiasm, energy, and interest in the subject to show

through body language. Appropriate gesticulation, facial gestures, and body movement add an element of theatrics to a presentation, focusing attention and increasing interest.

(b) Avoid physical habits which clearly distract from the presentation or limit its effectiveness (e.g., nose picking, hand over mouth, facing away from the audience, putting head down when talking).

(c) Avoid wearing clothing or equipment which unnecessarily obscures the face from the audience. Sunglasses are particularly distracting when they totally obscure eye contact.

c. **Methodology skills**
Selecting a method for presenting a lesson

(1) **Student knowledge**
How much do the students already know about the subject or skill? To what extent can they contribute to the lesson?

(2) **Student maturity**
How long is the group's attention span?

(3) **Student interest**
How much interest pre-exists in the subject or skill?

(4) **Time**
How much time is available for transmitting the essential information?

(5) **Nature of the subject**
Is the subject strictly a matter of fact, or is opinion or interpretation involved? How much emotional controversy may the subject potentially expose? Does discussion of the subject have the potential for negative impact on group morale? How abstract or concrete is the subject and what levels of intellectual ability will be expected of students for learning to take place?

4. **Lecture/demonstration**
  a. **Advantages of lecture/demonstration**
    (1) The maximum amount of factual or concrete information can be transmitted in the shortest amount of time.
    (2) Students need little or no pre-existing knowledge of the subject.
    (3) A controlled presentation of the material is guaranteed, limiting misunderstanding or misinterpretation of the instructor's statement.
    (4) It can be adapted to almost any environment.
    (5) It forces the group to focus on one specific topic or issue.
  b. **Disadvantages of lecture/demonstration**
    (1) It discourages a sense of active student intellectual or emotional involvement and participation in the learning process.
    (2) It does not generate a sense of emotional commitment to the outcome of the class.
    (3) The success or failure of the presentation is almost totally dependent upon the communication skills of the presenter.
    (4) It is very difficult to adequately determine varying degrees of cognitive ability in the audience.
  c. **Hints for success with lecture/demonstration**
    (1) The subject or skills should be narrowed down to the most important points. Keep it simple.
    (2) The method should be highly organized and logical, making note-taking easy.
    (3) A lecture should contain three distinct phases:
      (a) The introduction (tell 'em what you're gonna teach)
      (b) The body of knowledge (teach 'em)
      (c) The summary (tell 'em what you just taught 'em)
    (4) Use as many techniques as possible to expand student imagination. Use props — show as well as tell. Compare and contrast using common experience. Develop

appropriate metaphors. Illustrate with anecdotes.

(5) Be dramatic by using plenty of body movement, voice inflection, hand gesticulation, etc. Show emotion and use humor.

(6) Invite audience participation occasionally with direct questions, show of hands, or vocal acknowledgment.

(7) Keep it short. Read the audience for waning attention and either do something dramatic or give them a short break.

5. **Dialogue/discussion**

   a. **Advantages of dialogue/discussion**

(1) It is well-suited to development of abstract thoughts, opinions, attitudes, or judgment.

(2) It allows for individual development of higher levels of cognition such as analysis, synthesis, and evaluation.

(3) It encourages students to actively engage the mind and emotions in the learning process.

(4) It encourages students to be committed to their own learning.

(5) It allows students to thoroughly explore the subtleties and nuances of an idea or issue.

(6) The success of a class is not solely dependent on the presenter — students assume some responsibility and credit for the outcome.

(7) It may improve group morale if feelings and issues are revealed and resolved through group interaction.

   b. **Disadvantages of dialogue/discussion**

(1) It requires time. For participants to feel satisfied with the outcome, fruitful discussion shouldn't be rushed.

(2) It requires instructors to have very well-developed analytical skills in order to anticipate the flow of the discussion and keep it on track.

(3) It requires some pre-existing student knowledge of or opinion on the subject.

(4) Instructor objectives may not always be met by the discussion. It is more difficult

to control what specific knowledge is being transmitted.

(5) Discussion can lead to emotional confrontations that may require skillful conflict management to resolve.

(6) It requires extended periods of student attentiveness and patience while others express their views or opinions.

c. **Hints for success with dialogue/discussion**

(1) Always start with some specific and concrete issue, question, or statement. Move from the concrete to the abstract.

(2) The discussion leader should have some specific goals or knowledge which she or he wishes to have emerge. The leader should "guide" the discussion using skillful interrogation or comments. Sometimes it may be necessary to politely but firmly redirect the conversation to important points.

(3) The discussion leader should listen attentively, courteously, and empathetically to each student question or comment. It is important to not influence the group's response by indicating intolerance or disdain for the speaker.

(4) It is often necessary for the discussion leader to consciously divorce personal feelings from the discussion. Try to use non-judgmental language in dealing with student questions and responses.

(5) Invite participation from reticent group members by directly asking them questions to which they probably know the answer. After asking "confidence" questions, encourage broader, deeper thought.

(6) Help inarticulate group members to express their thoughts more clearly by rephrasing their statements after they speak, being cautious not to put words in their mouths.

(7) At the end of a discussion, clearly summarize the main points that were

reached so that all participants recognize the progress that was made.

d. **Skits**

Skits are an excellent tool to stimulate discussion.

(1) Be sure skit participants clearly understand the objectives of the skit. If necessary, write down the objectives.

(2) Pair less theatrical group members with one or two "hams" so that all students experience a comfortable sense of participation.

(3) Give all groups time to organize and practice their skit. Extemporaneous skits rarely provide enough substance for a quality discussion.

(4) Make sure that skit content is appropriate for the group. Avoid language or mannerisms that may mock specific group members.

(5) Encourage spontaneously creative scripts. Be careful of excessive slapstick which can become dangerous, hurtful, and distracting.

IV. **INSTRUCTIONAL STRATEGIES & MATERIALS:**

A. **Timing**

Although teaching techniques can be taught throughout the entire expedition, formal class presentations are usually most fruitful after instructors and students have both had the opportunity to experience some classes and compare instructor technique with student technique.

B. **Strategies**

1. This lesson is unique in that the very skill that is being taught must actually be used in organizing and presenting the subject. One of the most effective means of teaching this lesson is to point out good examples. Students should be encouraged to observe and analyze the techniques of instructors or other students whenever a "teaching" situation occurs. Such observations should be formally and informally discussed and analyzed for future use.

2. Whenever students are given the opportunity to "teach" a lesson, they should be encouraged to discuss their plans, techniques, and strategies with experienced instructors. Instructors should

encourage students to experiment with various techniques and strategies to find ones that suit the course. All student-taught lessons should be evaluated (either privately or in groups) in order to give immediate feedback.

3. Instructor-taught lessons should be models for various teaching techniques and strategies, and these classes should be evaluated in group sessions so that students understand the techniques used by the instructor. Instructors should be prepared to explain the rationale for their strategies, and also be willing to identify their own weaknesses so that students understand the need for constant self-evaluation in teaching.

C. **Activities**

The following activities have been used successfully in the field to illustrate various aspects of this lesson:

1. **Metaphor in teaching**

    a. Encourage participants to be creative in using their equipment or the resources of the natural environment as a metaphor to illustrate concepts.

    b. Camp gear can be used as a metaphor to illustrate teacher and student relationships.

        (1) **The teacher as a source of factual knowledge**

            Pour the contents of a filled water bottle into an empty cup to illustrate that, under certain circumstances, teachers "fill" their students with knowledge in order to give them necessary information. This metaphor might be used to introduce a discussion concerning the appropriate use of the lecture method.

        (2) **The teacher as a "spark" for new ideas and insights**

            Strike a wooden match against the abrasive surface of a matchbox to illustrate how a teacher may use the abrasive force of two minds rubbing together in heated dialogue or debate (the match and matchbox striking surface) to spark a new idea or perspective (the match flame). This

139

metaphor can introduce the appropriate
use of discussion/dialogue as a teaching tool.

(3) **The teacher as a beacon which shows the
way through example**
Use a flashlight to illustrate the way a
teacher can "enlighten" students by
helping them see better ways of doing things.

2. **Communication skills in teaching**

a. Participants should be encouraged to think up
games or activities that illustrate points they
wish to emphasize during a lesson. Activities
not only make an intellectual point, they also
break up a formal class with a refreshing
moment of productive fun and humor.

b. The "aardvark" activity may be used to
illustrate the fact that a teacher should use more
than just words to communicate an idea, since
the same word(s) may mean different things to
different people.

(1) Ask students to draw a picture of an object
which the instructor will describe. Ask
students not to collaborate on their
drawings or show their picture to anyone
else until it is completed.

(2) Tell students they are going to hear a
description of something and they should
draw a picture of what is described. The
students should add to their drawing as
each element of the description is read.

(3) Read the following description slowly,
phrase by phrase:

This "thing" weighs between 100 and 170
lbs. (45-77 kg.) and has a stout body that is
about 4 ft. long. It has a long tail (another 2
ft.) that is wider at the body and more
narrow at the tip. It has a narrow head
with a long snout, a long, slender tongue,
and no teeth in the front of the mouth. It
has donkey-like ears and short, thick legs
with partially webbed feet and strong,
blunt claws. This "thing" has a little bit of
hair on its body.

(4) Once students are finished drawing, compare the pictures to see how differently people interpreted the information. Use the activity to discuss methods that teachers can use other than words to communicate ideas and information (e.g., pictures, physical examples, skits, etc.).

c. **A "knotty" problem**

(1) In this exercise, participants are encouraged to consider the relationship between a particular subject or skill and the teaching method that is most appropriate to communicate it.

(2) In this exercise, the class is told that they will be taught a new knot. The class is going to be divided into three small groups with a different instructor teaching each group. At the end of the small group instruction, the entire class will be tested on their ability to tie the new knot.

(3) Each instructor will teach exactly the same knot using exactly the same directions to their small group. Only the method of teaching the knot will differ from group to group.

(4) Separate the three small groups so that they cannot see or hear the other groups. The students should have the illusion that they are all being taught the same way.

(5) **The directions**
The Improved Clinch Knot: Select a piece of rope at least two feet long. Loop the working end around a small tree or post. Take this same working end and circle it three times around the standing end of the rope. After completing these three circles, place the tip of the working end through the first loop formed by the crossing of the working and standing ends nearest the tree. Now take the tip of the working end and pass it through the loop you have just formed which is parallel to the standing

141

end. Pull the standing end of the rope to tighten the knot.

(a) **Group 1: lecture directions**
Slowly read the instructions to the group twice. Do not use any rope.

(b) **Group 2: lecture/demonstration directions**
Read the instructions and demonstrate the knot to the group. Do not let students touch the rope. Demonstrate it twice.

(c) **Group 3: group participation directions**
Give each student a piece of rope. While reading the directions, help each student tie the knot. Allow each student two opportunities to tie the knot.

(5) When the groups are finished with their lesson, have them come together for "testing." Have all students tie the knot simultaneously.

(6) In general, group 3 should do the best and group 1 the worst. Have the group sit down and discuss the results. "Process" the experience (as in a debriefing) until students discover the different teaching methods that were used with each group.

(7) Ask students to consider *why* some methods are more effective for teaching various types of subject and skills.

(8) Ask the group to discuss which teaching method they would use for each of the following: building a fire pit; the history of a local wilderness area; and the expedition behavior of a dishonest group member. Discuss the reasons students give for the methods they choose.

19. Trail Technique: Introductory

I. **GOAL:** To have participants understand the introductory concepts of trail technique so they may hike efficiently, comfortably, and safely while minimizing the chances of getting lost.

II. **OBJECTIVES:**
   A. Participants will understand the concept of energy conservation and why it is important.
   B. Participants will be able to practice the skill of rhythmic breathing.
   C. Participants will be able to follow a variety of different types of trails.
   D. Participants will be able to define the roles of scout, smoother, logger, and sweep.
   E. Participants will be able to understand the factors of pace, eating, clothing, and environmental awareness when hiking.
   F. Participants will understand the importance of group organization while hiking.

III. **CONTENT:**
   A. **The Energy Conservation Concept**
      1. **What is energy conservation?**
         a. The use of as little energy as possible to accomplish the task as efficiently and comfortably as possible (e.g., the tortoise and the hare).
         b. The concept involves coordinating the heartbeat and breathing to regulate the pace rather than the reverse (i.e., establish the pace, and then regulate heartbeat and breathing).
         c. The degree to which energy conservation should be practiced is related to the objectives of the outing (i.e., if physical challenge is a primary objective, then energy conservation techniques may be used less).

© 1992
The Wilderness Education Association
P.O. Box 89
Saranac Lake, New York 12983
(518) 891-2915 ext. 254

2. **What activities require energy conservation?**
   Any activity that requires above-average physical
   demands (e.g., high-altitude climbing, backpacking,
   day hiking, canoeing, kayaking, cross-country
   skiing, and snowshoeing)

3. **Why is it important to practice energy conservation?**
   a. Energy conservation minimizes changes in
      body temperature by decreasing perspiration.
   b. Elimination of fast starts and prolonged rests
      minimizes the fluctuation of heart beat rates.
   c. Increased endurance
      (1) Increased chance of arriving in camp
          without being exhausted
      (2) Energy is saved for emergency needs
      (3) Minimized chance of emotional outburst due
          to exhaustion and frustration
   d. Availability of less oxygen at higher altitudes
      may affect the brain, and therefore judgment.

4. **How are the components of energy conservation
   used?**
   a. **Rhythmic breathing**
      (1) Synchronize steps with breathing.
      (2) If breathing rate increases from increased
          effort, slow down the pace.
      (3) Develop a rhythm by coordinating the
          number of steps with the number of breaths.
          (a) On level terrain with a moderate load,
              take three large steps for every breath.
          (b) As the terrain gets steeper, the load
              heavier, or the oxygen thinner,
              shorten the step length and the
              number of breaths between steps.
      (4) The objective is to maintain a comfortable
          pace and still make forward progress.
      (5) With concentration and practice, rhythmic
          breathing will eventually become second
          nature.
   b. **Pace**
      (1) Pace is one of the most difficult things for
          a leader or scout to master. There is a
          tendency to hike too fast, which tires

144

group members. A good leader exhibits patience and has the ability to hike at a pace appropriate for the whole group.

(2) The pace is probably appropriate if:

    (a) A conversation can be held at all times while hiking.

    (b) The group can hike all day with occasional short rests and not be exhausted at the end of the day.

c. **Rest step**

The rest step is the point between steps where the skeletal structure provides support and gives the muscles a rest.

(1) Walk as flatfooted as possible, preventing the tiring of calf and foot muscles.

(2) Swing the foot up to the next step, lifting it no more than necessary. This saves on muscle exertion.

(3) Lock the knee with each step by putting weight on the skeletal system and not depending on the muscles for support.

(4) The steeper the terrain, the shorter the distance between steps and the longer the period of rest between steps.

(5) Dipping the shoulder on the side of the lead foot takes the weight of the pack off that shoulder, allowing it to rest.

d. **Rest breaks**

(1) The objective should be resting to *prevent* exhaustion not *because of* exhaustion.

(2) If it is difficult to make it from rest break to rest break, either:

    (a) The pace is too fast

    (b) The time between breaks is too long

(3) How often and for how long should the group break?

    (a) Establish hiking/resting times (e.g., hike 30 minutes, rest 5) and stick to them for a couple of hours; modify if necessary.

    (b) Be sure to communicate to the group what the break times will be and stick to them. This gives weaker members of the group a goal to work towards and something to look forward to.

(c) Depending on factors such as the group's physical condition, trip objectives, and the hiking terrain, hiking and resting times range from hiking 20 minutes and resting 5, to hiking an hour and resting 5 to 10 minutes. Again, remember to rest before becoming tired, not when the group is already tired.

(4) **Length of break**
Five minute breaks will minimize lactic acid buildup, a waste product of muscle activity. While this is a worthy goal, it is difficult to achieve. Whatever length of time is decided on, try to stick to it unless judgment dictates otherwise.

(5) **Where to break**
(a) Have the scout pick a site that is reasonably comfortable with an available water source. It is usually worth hiking an extra ten minutes or taking a break five minutes early to have a good rest break location.

(b) Have the group rest on one side of the trail and well out of the way of others who may come down the trail.

(6) **Starting and ending the break**
(a) Start the break when the last person gets to the break location.

(b) Be sure to communicate clearly how long the break will be.

(c) Announce to the group when one minute is left. Be sure the group understands that they should start putting on packs at this time.

(7) **Eating and drinking at breaks**
Encourage the intake of fluids and calories during breaks to replenish lost water and burned up energy.

(8) **Flexibility**
Be sure to remain flexible. If a break needs
to be taken early, take it. If the group
needs extra time, give it to them. Don't be
so tied to a schedule that the fun is taken
out of the hike.

B. **Trail Hiking**
1. **Tips for following marked trails**
    a. Understand the importance of knowing where
        the group is at all times. Make sure the trail
        goes where it is expected to go. Keep
        comparing the map with the terrain.
    b. Learn to follow trail markers, blazes, and
        cairns. (Cairns are piles of rocks that mark a
        trail.) Trails can give a false sense of security
        and may not go where expected.
        (1) A season's growth of vegetation may
             cover up trail blazes.
        (2) Missing just one marker can be misleading
             and throw hikers off a marked trail.
2. **Tips for following rarely-hiked trails**
    a. Pay careful attention to map, compass, and
        terrain, since the trail may be overgrown with
        vegetation and not clearly identifiable.
    b. Watch carefully for trail markers, since they
        may be covered or missing.
3. **Trail courtesy**
    a. Move to one side and let other groups go by.
    b. Come to a complete stop and stand to the
        downhill side when encountering horses.
        Horses are very easily spooked by humans
        wearing backpacks. Speak softly to the horse
        packers and make the horses aware of the
        group's presence.

C. **Miscellaneous Hiking Considerations**
1. **Hiking uphill**
    a. Stand straight to maintain balance or improve
        the chances of being able to recover quickly if

footing is lost. Use the rest step as described earlier in this lesson.

    b.   Smaller steps conserve energy.

    c.   If obstacles are too large to step over easily, go around them.

2. **Hiking downhill**

    a.   Injuries may be more likely to occur while walking downhill.

    b.   Bend the knees slightly and use small, controlled steps to help resist the force of gravity that pulls the body forward.

    c.   Try different ways of tying boots to help minimize friction and maximize comfort.

3. **Contouring**

    a.   A less direct route with fewer elevation changes will help conserve energy, and may also be easier and safer.

    b.   Judgment should determine whether contouring is the best option.

4. **Clothing**

Rest breaks should be used to add or shed clothing and maintain a constant and comfortable body temperature. (See "Clothing Selection" lesson for a more detailed discussion of climate control.)

5. **Low impact considerations**

    a.   **Walking along the trail**

       If at all possible, do not widen the treadway if the trail is muddy.

    b.   **Human waste disposal along the trail**

       Along the trail, hikers should dispose of waste in catholes using the same guidelines as those discussed in the "Latrine Construction and Use" lesson.

    c.   **Trail litter**

       In addition to packing out whatever was brought in, participants should be encouraged to pack out any other litter that is found along the trail. This is a good way to express stewardship and avoid hypocritical practices. This issue can be further addressed in the

"Environmental Ethics and Backcountry
Conservation Practices" lesson.

D. **Trail Logistics and Organization**
    1. **Assigning trail responsibilities**
        Stress the importance of trail organization. Split-up
        groups that can't communicate are a contributing
        cause of lost hikers.
    2. **Group size**
        Optimal group size should be determined using the
        following considerations:
        a. **Safety**
            How many people can be safely organized and
            monitored?
        b. **Environmental impact**
            What group size will have the least amount of
            impact on the area?
        c. **Social carrying capacity**
            What group size will have minimal aesthetic
            and psychological impact on the group and
            other users?
        d. **Managing agency policies**
            Does the managing agency have regulations
            that will determine or influence group size?
    3. **Group roles**
        a. **Leader**
            The leader may want to travel back and forth
            among the group to stay aware of how
            participants are feeling. The leader has overall
            responsibility for the group and ultimate
            decision-making responsibility.
            (1) The leader may determine:
                (a) Rest stop times and locations (with
                    the logger's input)
                (b) Lunch stop time and location
                (c) When and where the campsite should
                    be established
            (2) Stress the importance of communication
                between the leader and the group.
        b. **Scout**
            The scout sets the pace and consults with the
            leader to determine the route. The scout is
            obviously at the front of the line.

149

c. **Smoother**

When hiking off-trail, the smoother improves the route which the scout selects.

   (1) The smoother must stay far enough behind the scout to make this effective.

   (2) Judgment can dictate when and where a smoother is necessary.

   d. **Logger**

   (1) The logger notes all times of the day's activities.

   (2) This information can be used to develop future "Time Control Plans."

   (3) Generally, these times are reviewed during debriefings. The logger is responsible for having the times available at debriefings.

   e. **Sweep**

The sweep is the last person in line.

   (1) The sweep makes sure no one gets behind and that the pace is appropriate for the group.

   (2) The sweep makes sure the group does not get too spread out.

   (3) The sweep should communicate with the scout and leader in particular.

IV. **INSTRUCTIONAL STRATEGIES & MATERIALS:**

   Timing

   1. An introduction and overview of the topics in this lesson are appropriate on a morning early in the trip. Most of the material can be taught and reinforced on the trail using "teachable moments."

   2. Debriefings are an important means of reinforcing these concepts and gaining an indication of how well participants understand them and can practice them. The importance of debriefing the previous day's trail experiences cannot be over-emphasized.

20. Trail Technique: Advanced

I. **GOAL**: To have participants understand the advanced concepts of trail technique so they may hike efficiently, comfortably, and safely while minimizing the chances of getting lost.

II. **OBJECTIVES**:
   A. Participants will be able to deal with situations and concerns that arise on the trail.
   B. Participants will understand how to avoid blisters and care for them while hiking.
   C. Participants will be able to make a "Time Control Plan" based on a variety of considerations.
   D. Participants will understand the importance of physical fitness in making a hike enjoyable and safe.
   E. Participants will understand the importance of knowing their approximate location at all times.

III. **CONTENT**:
   A. **Slower hikers**
      1. If the weakest or slowest hikers are left at the end of the group to constantly worry about catching up, it will likely have a negative psychological effect on them.
      2. Try putting slower hikers near the front of the group and have the scout set a pace that they can keep up with. Try having slower hikers scout.
         a. The responsibility of being scout will take their mind off the physical effort of the hike.
         b. Eliminating weight from a weaker hiker's pack may enable them to travel a bit faster. This should be offered diplomatically to avoid hurt feelings.
         c. Help slower hikers by providing encouragement, or engaging them in conversation or activities to take their mind off the physical effort. Remind them that they will get stronger as the days go by.

© 1992
The Wilderness Education Association
P.O. Box 89
Saranac Lake, New York 12983
(518) 891-2915 ext. 254

B.   The "Time Control Plan
"Time Control Plans" (TCP's) take into account terrain, distance, altitude, group objectives, trail conditions, and the group's condition to determine how long it will take to reach a destination. They usually include hiking times, rest times, and total travel time.

1.   **Knowing the country**
It is important to know the country well. If this is not possible, be conservative in planning.

2.   **Flexibility**
Once a plan has been developed and is instituted, be sure to continuously reevaluate progress and, if necessary, modify the objectives. If progress is not satisfactory, don't be afraid to turn back.

3.   **Building on experience**
As you gain experience in wilderness travel, use that experience in developing the "TCP."

C.   **Blister Prevention and Care**
1.   **Prevention**
   a.   **Socks**
      (1)   Wearing two pair of socks will help minimize blisters, which are caused by the friction of a boot or sock against the foot. Two socks will rub against each other and the boot, minimizing friction against the foot.
      (2)   Adjusting socks and boot laces can help prevent blisters or minimize discomfort once they develop.
   b.   **Walking technique**
   Walking flat-footed will also help minimize blisters because the foot will do less bending, thereby generating less friction.
   c.   **Hot spots**
   It is important to stop and care for feet before a blister occurs. Learn to feel hot spots and take preventive measures without delay.
   d.   **Feet**
      (1)   Applying moleskin at the trailhead may prevent further troubles down the trail.

(2) Use of foot powder or vaseline on the feet can also help prevent blisters.

  e. **Checking on the group**
   Leaders should frequently check with the group to see how their feet are doing during the early part of the trip. In some cases, foot checks in which all hikers bare their feet for inspection may be necessary.

 2. **Care**
  Moleskin, molefoam, Second Skin™
  a. Use on hot spots.
  b. Use once a blister has formed.
  c. Moleskin reduces friction and, because it is thin, fits easily inside a boot.
  d. Molefoam provides more cushioning but may take up more room inside a boot because it is thicker.
  e. Second Skin™ is a thin layer of gel that has a cooling effect on hot spots and blisters, relieving soreness. It practically eliminates friction. However, it is a more expensive alternative and additional tape is necessary to apply it because it has no adhesive.

D. **Trailless Hiking**
 1. **Thick forest cover**
  a. Everyone has the responsibility to stay a safe distance behind the person in front of them so they don't get a branch slapped in their face.
  b. Minimize the "accordion effect" by being sure the group does not get too spread out.
  c. Hikers will cause less environmental impact by spreading out on a trailless hike rather than walking in a straight line.
   (1) This minimizes the impact caused by several feet trampling the same vegetation.
   (2) This minimizes the chance of starting a new trail.
  d. Be careful of what may be beneath thick vegetation and brush. There may be holes, streams, rocks, or other hazards below.

 2. **Use of game trails**
  a. Game trails are natural trails formed by animals traveling through the area.

b.   They often provide the best route when hiking off-trail, since they usually follow a path of least resistance.

     c.   It is still advisable to keep track of the route with map and compass, since the path may not lead to the group's destination.

  3. **Talus and scree slopes**
Talus and scree are rock fragments that have broken off cliffs or peaks.

     a.   Talus ranges in size from rocks the size of cobblestones to small boulders. Talus is often sharp-edged, making falls dangerous.

        (1)   Descending talus slopes can be more difficult than ascending, since downward momentum increases the risk of falling more often and further.

        (2)   Hiking on talus requires precise footing and quick, light steps to move from rock to rock.

     b.   Scree ranges from the size of sand to the size of a fist. Ascending scree is more difficult than descending because it slips easily underfoot.

     c.   Keep the group close together on either talus or scree so that rocks that are loosened by one hiker don't pick up too much speed before hitting the next hiker.

     d.   Group members should avoid walking beneath the fall line of those ahead in case rocks are loosened.

     e.   If a rock is loosened and/or falls, hikers should shout "Rock!" to warn those below of the danger.

E. **The Role of Physical Fitness**

  1. **Values of physical fitness**

     a.   Being physically fit allows for more enjoyment because fatigue doesn't occur as quickly.

     b.   It helps to minimize frustration and interpersonal conflict.

     c.   It avoids injuries and illnesses.

     d.   It provides an extra margin of safety in emergency situations.

  2. **The importance of physical fitness for the leader**

     a.   The leader has a responsibility to be at least as physically fit as the average person in the group, and preferably to be as fit as the strongest person in the group.

b.   This allows the leader to plan and lead trips that are physically challenging for the whole group.

c.   Individuals paying for a wilderness experience have a right to expect their leader to be physically fit.

d.   A fit leader insures an extra margin of safety in case of emergency.

IV. INSTRUCTIONAL STRATEGIES & MATERIALS:

A.   **Timing**
This lesson should be taught after participants have gained some experience on the trail by using teachable moments (e.g., when a participant gets a blister).

B.   **Activities**

1.   **"Time Control Plans"**

a.   It is recommended that each participant write up a TCP on a daily basis and hand it in to the LOD.

b.   At the next debriefing, the TCP's are compared to the logger's official times.

c.   This activity allows participants to start creating an experience base which can aid in estimating how long a given trip will take.

d.   This activity can be turned into a game with a prize given to the individual with the most accurate TCP.

2.   **Contour counting**

a.   Each morning before participants write up their TCP, one participant is asked to count the contours to the destination.

b.   The individual counts each contour as either an "up contour" or a "down contour."

c.   The logger keeps a count and adds up the total number of "up contours" and the total number of "down contours."

d.   The elevation of feet the group will ascend and descend is then used as an aid in computing the TCP.

e.   This activity accomplishes two objectives:
- (1) It develops map reading skills.
- (2) It stresses the role that elevation change has in determining how long it takes to get to the group's destination.

C. **Materials**
1. Maps (at least one for every two people)
2. Moleskin and molefoam
3. Second Skin™
4. Scissors
5. Pencil or pen
6. Paper

21. Trip Planning

I. **GOAL:** To have participants understand how to plan safe, enjoyable, and environmentally sound wilderness trips of various lengths.

II. **OBJECTIVES:**
   A. Participants will be able to list and explain guidelines of trip planning.
   B. Participants will be able to list and explain various considerations in planning a trip.

III. **CONTENT:**
   A. **Trip Planning Guidelines**
      1. **Organization**
         Use an organizational structure so group members know who they are responsible to and what their responsibilities are.
      2. **Lists**
         Make lists and utilize them. Possible lists include:
         a. Things to do
         b. Things to buy
         c. Equipment and clothing
         d. Food
         e. Recommendations for future trips
      3. **Anticipate**
         Plan ahead and anticipate what may happen and what can be done. Have contingency plans. For example, what will be done if certain equipment doesn't arrive in time?

   B. **Trip Planning Considerations**
      1. **Goals and objectives**
         a. Without clear group objectives, individuals seek personal objectives which may clash and result in an unsuccessful trip or even disaster.

b. Insuring that everyone knows and agrees to the trip objectives contributes to the success of the trip. Once an individual agrees to the trip objectives, that person then has a vested interest and a responsibility to see that objectives are met.

2. **Leadership**
  a. Are there qualified people making decisions?
  b. Is a feeling of trust, comfort, and safety communicated by those in the leadership role?
  c. Is there someone assuming overall responsibility for what happens?

3. **Itinerary**
  The itinerary should be made in conjunction with:
  a. Trip objectives
  b. Physical abilities and limitations of group members

4. **Emergency planning** (see "Emergency Planning" and "Risk Management" lessons)
  Develop a plan which includes:
  a. Preventive measures
  b. Emergency procedures in an emergency situation
  c. Evacuation options
  d. Post-emergency plans

5. **Liability**
  a. Does the program have an overall risk management plan?
  b. Is there adequate liability insurance coverage?
  c. Is there an assumption of risk form?
   (1) Waiver of claims
   (2) Liability releases
  d. Do participants have accident and illness insurance?

6. **Land management rules and regulations**
  a. Is there knowledge of rules and regulations?
  b. Are permits needed, where is camping legal, etc.?

7. **Food and nutrition** (see "Nutrition and Rations Planning" lesson)
  a. How will food be selected?
  b. How will amounts and nutritional balance be determined?
  c. Who will purchase and pack food?
  d. How will food drops be coordinated?

8. **Equipment and clothing** (see "Clothing Selection" lesson)
    a. Develop a master equipment and clothing list.
    b. What needs to be purchased?
    c. Who is responsible for clothing and equipment acquisition?
    d. How and when will equipment and clothing be issued?
9. **Skills and knowledge**
    a. What skills and knowledge do individuals have?
    b. What skills and topics should be reviewed before the trip?
    c. Who will teach specific skills and topics during the trip?
10. **Expedition behavior**
    What steps have been taken to insure that group members will get along and that objectives can be met?
11. **Water sources**
    Where is potable water available?
12. **Finances**
    a. Is there a budget?
    b. Who is responsible for the expenses and how much money is needed?
    c. Who will handle the finances and how will it be documented?
13. **Weather**
    a. What are the historical weather patterns in the area?
    b. What is the short-term weather forecast?
    c. What is the long-term weather forecast?
    d. Who will keep a log of the weather during the trip?
14. **Transportation**
    a. Who will provide vehicles?
    b. What are vehicles needed for specifically?
        (1) Shopping
        (2) Transportation to and from the trailhead
        (3) Laundry after the trip
    c. Are they in properly-maintained condition?
    d. Who is responsible for the cost of the vehicles (e.g., fuel, oil, and maintenance)?
    e. Who will drive the vehicles?

f. Will drivers know when and where to meet the group, and the route and destination?

15. **Resources**

  a. **Human**

  Is there anyone who has been to the planned trip area before who can give you first-hand information (e.g., rangers, locals, guides, etc.)?

  b. **Written**

  Are there books, brochures, magazine articles, or other written materials available about the area?

  c. **Photographic**

  Are there photographs available of the area?

  d. **Maps**

  Are there new or old maps available of the area?

16. **Post trip**

  a. Are shower facilities available?

  b. Where and when will the group debrief the overall trip, and when will student and course evaluations take place?

  c. Who will inventory the leftover food?

  d. Where and when will the group do laundry?

  e. How will equipment be repaired and inventoried?

  f. Who will write thank-you notes for anyone who helped out?

  g. Who will make arrangements for a party or banquet?

  h. How will extra food and equipment be disposed of?

17. **Public relations**

  a. Who will arrange for press releases for participants' home town newspapers?

  b. Who will organize photographs for press releases and future promotion?

  c. Will t-shirts, patches, pins, and other memorabilia be available for group participants or for fund-raising?

IV. **INSTRUCTIONAL STRATEGIES & MATERIALS:**

 A. **Timing**

  When this lesson is taught is dependent on whether or to what extent participants are involved in the planning of the course. If participants are involved in the actual planning of the trip, then this becomes a high priority lesson at the outset. If participants are not involved in the planning of the trip, then this becomes a lower priority lesson which can be taught later in the course.

B. **Strategies**

Different WEA affiliates involve participants in trip planning to varying degrees. Options include:

1. Having participants plan nearly every aspect of the expedition.
2. Having participants get involved in certain aspects of the expedition (e.g., food planning and itinerary).
3. Having participants not get involved in the direct planning of their WEA course but get involved in subsequent expeditions. At North Country Community College for example, participants have little involvement in planning their WEA course but have nearly total responsibility for planning a subsequent two-week winter expedition.

C. **Activities**

Have participants get involved in specific phases of trip planning (whether a short trip or an extended trip). It is important to evaluate their planning process and give them specific feedback.

22. Water Safety

by Brian McDonnell

I. **GOAL**: To have participants be aware of and use swimming and canoeing safety practices.

II. **OBJECTIVES**:
- A. Participants will be able to identify an appropriate swim site.
- B. Participants will be able to check a site for obstructions.
- C. Participants will be able to identify swimming abilities.
- D. Participants will be able to put on a personal flotation device (PFD) in deep water.

III. **CONTENTS**
- A. **Water Safety**
  1. **Why practice water safety?**
     - a. It is better to be "safe than sorry."
     - b. Water safety practices reduce overall risk of the trip.
     - c. Evacuation could take several days, can be costly, and could even end an expedition.
  2. **Selecting a swim site**
     - a. The needs of the group should be considered when selecting a swim site. Some examples include:
       - (1) A group of non-swimmers would be uncomfortable in a pool that is 10 ft. (3 m.) deep with rock sidewalls.
       - (2) It would not be appropriate for a group of strong swimmers to be limited to waist-high water.

b. An ideal swim site would be sandy, gradually sloping, clear of glass, trees, and vegetation and with no strong current. However, such a site is rarely found in the wilderness.

c. Inspecting potential swim sites is an important precaution and should not be overlooked.

3. **Inspecting the site**

a. Before allowing anyone to enter a swimming area, check the site for obstructions.

b. Rocks, logs, broken glass, fish hooks, and sudden dropoffs are all potential hazards.

4. **Identifying swimming ability**

a. At the first opportunity, the trip leader or assigned waterfront safety person should identify the swimming ability of each group member. A simple 100 yard swim followed by a 3 minute float will allow the leader to determine adequate swimming ability.

b. Identifying swimming ability gives the leader an opportunity to offer instruction to weaker swimmers.

5. **Adequate supervision**

a. Someone with knowledge of reaching and throwing rescue techniques and the potential hazards of a swim area should be assigned to supervise any swimming activity.

b. This "lifeguard" should know how many people are in the water at all times. One method is to have swimmers leave a shirt or sneaker in a designated place while they are in the water. The number of shirts or sneakers would correspond with the number of swimmers in the water.

c. A moonlit swim can be a refreshing sensory experience, but the added dimension of darkness can lead to disorientation. Adequate supervision and judgment are necessary to conduct safe activities.

6. **Adequate knowledge**

a. Make no assumptions. Observe each participant's swimming ability.

b. Anyone leading groups in, on, or around water should be skilled in lifesaving techniques.

c.   Identify hazards and take steps to avoid problems (e.g., mark hazards and have participants wear sneakers in the water if there is any risk of broken glass, shells, or other hazardous objects).

      d.   Stay well away from water during lightning storms — water is a great conductor of electricity.

B.   **Canoe Safety**
    1.   **Canoeing safety standards**
        a.   Check the load capacity of the canoe and don't exceed it.
        b.   Canoes will handle most efficiently when they are level on the water, or "trimmed" correctly. All cargo should be below the gunwales of the canoe and resting on the bottom, if possible. If gear is piled above the gunwales, the canoe will be less stable.
        c.   Paddling partners can be determined by matching physical size and canoeing ability (e.g., match those of similar size and weight but match less skilled paddlers with skilled paddlers).

    2.   **Personal flotation devices (PFD's)**
        a.   Inspect all PFD's. Make sure there are no tears and PFD's are serviceable.
        b.   Make sure PFD's fit participants properly and comfortably.
        c.   PFD's should be worn by weak swimmers at all times, and by all group members when deemed necessary by the group leader (e.g., windy, cold, whitewater, choppy conditions).
           (1)   Some agencies have established policies that dictate who should wear PFD's and when.
           (2)   Essentially, the issue of who should wear PFD's and when represents the WEA philosophy..."rules are for fools." It is a controversial issue that is often governed by rules, but ultimately one in which judgment should determine when PFD's are necessary.

d. PFD's should be in a "ready-to-use" condition and location when they are not being worn.

e. A safety drill might include putting PFD's on in the water and also jumping into the water with PFD's on. The purpose of this is to check the fit and get the feel of wearing a PFD in water.

3. **Canoes**

a. Even when trimmed correctly, canoes can capsize. Canoes are designed to provide adequate buoyancy to float even when they are full of water.

b. Canoes can be righted and paddled or swum to shore even with a full load of water.

c. **Canoe rescues**

(1) After a canoe has capsized, the safety of the paddlers should be of prime concern.

(a) Check to see if they are hurt.

(b) Check for signs of immersion hypothermia.

i) If the sum of the air temperature and the water temperature is less than 100, hypothermia is a potential danger.

ii) Someone who has been in water that is 50° F or less for 20 minutes or more will be suffering from a severe amount of heat loss.

(c) Be sure they are wearing PFD's.

(2) If there is no danger of hypothermia and the paddlers are wearing PFD's and have adjusted to being in the water, a second canoe may assist in righting the capsized craft.

(3) **Canoe-over-canoe rescue**

(a) If gear remains in the capsized boat, it should be taken out before attempting a rescue. Any gear that has gone overboard can be collected by other group members.

(b) The victims should assist the rescue boat by bringing the capsized canoe to a "T" at the midship of the rescue

canoe. With this accomplished, the
victims should go to either end of the
rescue canoe and hold on.

(4) The rescuers then pull the swamped vessel
over their canoe, empty the water, and
return it to the water right side up.

(5) The rescuers can then assist the victims by
holding their craft, enabling them to climb
back in (either one at a time or both at once
on opposite sides of the canoe).

IV. INSTRUCTIONAL STRATEGIES & MATERIALS:

A. Timing

1. A pre-trip discussion of safety considerations is
advisable.

2. At the first swim site, demonstrate the process for
selecting a proper swim area to show the safety
considerations that are involved.

B. Strategies

1. A "teachable moment" can be used to instruct
proper canoe loading and unloading techniques,
and should accompany this lesson.

2. PFD's should be serviceable and fitted before the
trip departs.

3. Participants can practice canoe-over-canoe rescues
during the trip.

C. Activities

1. Ask students to discuss specific safety
considerations.

2. Assign a different person each day to be responsible
for swim site selection.

3. Include safety concerns as part of daily debriefings.
Were there any potential problems?

4. A canoe race during which participants capsize
boats, put on PFD's, and paddle back to shore is an
effective teaching technique. Be sure to have a safety
boat standing by.

23. Water Treatment

I. **GOAL:** To have participants understand when, why, and how to treat water.

II. **OBJECTIVES:**
   A. Participants will be able to explain when water should be treated.
   B. Participants will be able to explain why water should be treated.
   C. Participants will be able to describe three methods of water treatment and demonstrate one of those methods.

III. **CONTENT:**
   A. **When Should Water be Treated?**
      1. Whenever there is any doubt about water purity.
      2. Due to the presence of pathogenic bacteria, protozoans, and enteroviruses throughout the world, there are few places totally free of contaminants.
      3. It should be understood that consuming untreated water is a gamble — be prepared to pay the price!

   B. **Why Does Water Have to be Treated?**
      1. **Bacterial and protozoan pathogens**
         a. These are single-cell organisms capable of causing disease that are present in all water.
         b. There are many different pathogens, but a common one is Giardia lamblia.
            (1) Giardia lamblia is a protozoan.
            (2) It is one of the most identifiable problems in wilderness water consumption today.
            (3) It is a parasite that causes the gastrointestinal illness Giardiasis.
            (4) It occurs throughout the United States.

© 1992
The Wilderness Education Association
P.O. Box 89
Saranac Lake, New York 12983
(518) 891-2915 ext. 254

(5) Symptoms of Giardiasis include:
  (a) Diarrhea
  (b) Abdominal cramps
  (c) Flatulence
  (d) Nausea
  (e) An eventual nutritional deficiency due to malabsorption of nutrients

 (6) **Diagnosis and treatment**
  (a) Diagnosis is through examination of fecal smears.
  (b) It is most commonly treated with drugs such as quinicrine, metronidazole, furazolidone and tinidazole.

 (7) **Other facts about Giardia**
  (a) Giardia is carried and spread by all mammals (not just beaver).
  (b) One stool can contain up to three hundred million cysts, which are infectious forms of Giardia.
  (c) Ingesting as few as ten cysts can cause the disease.
  (d) The length of illness ranges from a few days to three months.
  (e) Most infected individuals (75%) experience no symptoms and never realize they have had it (Bloch & Patzkowsky, 1985).
  (f) All backpackers must consider themselves carriers of Giardiasis and dispose of their human waste appropriately. (See "Latrine Construction and Use" lesson.)
  (g) Should symptoms of diarrhea, flatulence, and/or nausea persist, a physician should be consulted.

 (8) Some noted physicians feel Giardiasis is blown out of proportion because:
  (a) Most people won't even know they have ingested cysts.
  (b) A few people will get an intestinal upset similar to a nasty hangover.

(c) Fewer still will get a troublesome illness which responds well to therapy.

(d) As one doctor put it, "This...places Giardiasis in the category of blisters and mosquito bites: a nuisance reminder of a trip in the wilderness for some, with an occasional hiker developing a more serious complication" (Welch, 1986).

(9) **Legal implications**
Although the chances of a participant getting seriously ill are remote, trip leaders may be considered negligent if no preventative measures are taken.

2. **Enteroviruses (intestinal viruses)**
   a. They are simpler and generally smaller than bacteria.
   b. The symptoms may be treated, but generally the body's immune system eliminates them.
   c. Human viruses can only come from other humans, and therefore only spread as a result of human contamination.
   d. Enterovirus symptoms are similar to Giardia, but are usually short-lived.
   e. Enteroviruses may be considered less of a concern than other pathogens when backpacking in North America because of their short-term effect on the digestive system. However, the symptoms are still very discomforting.

C. **Methods of Treating Water**
1. **Boiling**
   a. Microorganisms such as Giardia, viruses, and harmful bacteria are sensitive to heat.
   b. Various sources recommend conflicting times and temperatures for heating water. The range includes:
      (1) Temperatures: 122° F (50° C) - 212° F (100°C)
      (2) Times: 0-15 minutes at these temperatures.

c.   Research indicates that water which reaches a full boil is safe to drink. Additional boiling time is **not** necessary.

    d.   **Advantages of boiling**

        (1)   It is inexpensive — the only expense is the fuel.

        (2)   It is completely effective when the water reaches a full boil.

        (3)   Boiling does not affect the taste of the water.

    e.   **Disadvantages of boiling**

        (1)   It takes time and consumes fuel.

        (2)   It is inconvenient for drinking water along the trail.

2. **Filtration**

    a.   Filters are commercially available that will filter out Giardia and bacteria. Some filters will even filter out large viruses.

    b.   Filters must trap particles at least as small as 0.5 microns.

    c.   **Advantages of filtration**

        (1)   It is easy to filter drinking water along the trail.

        (2)   Filtration does not affect the taste of the water.

    d.   **Disadvantages of filtration**

        (1)   Filters are generally slow (1-3 minutes per liter).

        (2)   Filters are often ineffective against entero-viruses.

        (3)   Filtration is a more expensive method due to the cost of filters ($30-$175).

3. **Chemical treatment**

    a.   **Crystalline iodination**
       Commercial brands are available such as "Polar Pure."

        (1)   A small amount of water is added to an iodine solution. After this water is disinfected (how long it takes depends on water temperature) the solution is added to a larger water source to achieve a final concentration of saturated iodine solution.

(2) **Advantages of crystalline iodination**
   (a) If used correctly, it is completely effective.
   (b) It is inexpensive.
   (c) It is easy to use.
   (d) Its shelf life is unlimited.

(3) **Disadvantages of crystalline iodination**
   (a) Water must sit for 30 minutes or longer (up to several hours if it is cold water) before consumption.
   (b) It has some effect on the taste of the water.
   (c) As with any chemical, large concentrated doses have the potential to be toxic.

b. **Iodine tablets**
Commercial brands are available such as "Potable Aqua" or "Globaline."

(1) A tablet which releases an iodine solution is added directly to the water.

(2) **Advantages of iodine**
   (a) It is readily available.
   (b) It is easy to use.
   (c) If used properly, it is usually effective.

(3) **Disadvantages of iodine**
   (a) Water must sit for 30 minutes or longer (up to several hours if it is cold water) before consumption.
   (b) Iodine affects the taste of the water.
   (c) Tablets have a limited shelf life and lose effectiveness from frequent exposure to air.
   (d) As with any chemical, large concentrated doses have the potential to be toxic.

c. **Chlorination**
Commercial brands are available such as "Halazone" tablets.

(1) **Advantages of chlorination**
   (a) It is readily available.
   (b) It is inexpensive.
   (c) It is easy to use.

(2) **Disadvantages of chlorination**

   (a) It is not always effective against Giardia lamblia (.5% chlorine concentrations commonly used by municipal water systems do not assure effectiveness).

   (b) Water must sit for 30 minutes or longer (up to several hours if it is cold water) before consumption.

   (c) Chlorine affects the taste of the water.

   (d) "Halazone" has a shelf life of 5 months if it is stored at 89° F (32° C). Its effectiveness is reduced if it is stored at higher temperatures or exposed to air.

   (e) As with any chemical, large concentrated doses have the potential to be toxic.

IV. INSTRUCTIONAL STRATEGIES & MATERIALS:

A. **Timing**

This topic should be introduced immediately and course policy communicated as to what types of treatment will be used.

B. **Strategies**

1. It is essential that if water is to be treated, instructors set a consistent example.

2. When teaching this class, it is important to demonstrate at least one means of water treatment.

  a. Filtration or chemical treatment are preferable methods of water treatment to demonstrate.

  b. Use the water source as a classroom setting and demonstrate the whole sequence from water acquisition to treatment and consumption.

C. **Materials**

1. Equipment for at least one type of water treatment

2. Water container

3. Water source (stream, lake, or spring)

24. WEA History

The authors would like to recognize Dr. Frank Lupton as a major contributor to this chapter.

I.   **GOAL**: To have participants understand and explain the evolution and basic philosophy of the Wilderness Education Association.

II. **OBJECTIVES**:
   A.   Participants will be able to explain the historical linkage between the Wilderness Education Association (WEA), the National Outdoor Leadership School (NOLS), and Outward Bound (OB), and describe the philosophies of each.
   B.   Participants will be able to describe the chronological history of the WEA.
   C.   Participants will be able to explain the WEA mission statement and WEA's niche in the education system.
   D.   Participants will be able to identify the 18 points of the WEA curriculum.
   E.   Participants will be able to list and describe the various levels of WEA certification.
   F.   Participants will be able to describe the relationship between the WEA and its affiliates.
   G.   Participants will be able to list eight WEA affiliates.

III. **CONTENT**:
   A.   **History and philosophy of WEA, NOLS, and OB**
       1.   Paul Petzoldt's career in wilderness education is the common thread that binds these three international organizations.
           a.   An internationally recognized pioneer in the field of wilderness education, Paul's early exploits provided the experience and back-

© 1992
The Wilderness Education Association
P.O. Box 89
Saranac Lake, New York 12983
(518) 891-2915 ext. 254

ground which became the foundation of his
later teachings.

   b. Petzoldt directed the Petzoldt-Exum School of
American Mountaineering in the Teton Range
during the 1920s.

   c. He was a member of the first American expedition to K2 in the Himalaya in 1938.

   d. He taught mountain evacuation and cold-weather
dress to U.S. ski troops during World War II.

   e. He is the author of *The New Wilderness Handbook*.

2. **Outward Bound (OB)**

   a. Conceived by Kurt Hahn, "Outward Bound
grew out of the need to instill a spiritual
tenacity and the will to survive in young British
seamen being torpedoed by German U-boats
during World War II. What began as a training
exercise for apprentice British seamen and
youth in Wales has since evolved into a modern-
day program for self-discovery and personal
development" (Outward Bound, 1987, p. 4).

   b. Outward Bound was brought to North America in
1963 by Josh Miner who hired Paul Petzoldt as
Chief Instructor for the Colorado Outward
Bound School.

   c. Outward Bound operates from five established
schools around the country.

   d. **The Outward Bound Philosophy**
"...Outward Bound's purpose is to develop and
enhance in its participants self-confidence and
self-esteem, leadership, teamwork and empathy
for others" (Outward Bound, 1987, p. 4).

3. **National Outdoor Leadership School (NOLS)**

   a. Frustrated by the lack of qualified instructors in
the profession, and responding to the growing
public interest in backcountry travel, Paul
Petzoldt founded the National Outdoor
Leadership School in 1965.

   b. **The NOLS Mission statement**
"...to be the best source and teacher of
wilderness skills and leadership which protect
the user and the environment" (National Outdoor
Leadership School, 1991, p. 3).

c.   NOLS operates from established bases located around the world.

4.   **Wilderness Education Association (WEA)**

    a.   In 1976, a group of Western Illinois University students led by Paul Petzoldt and Dr. Frank Lupton traveled through the Targhee National Forest of Wyoming and the Wind River Range on an experimental course which would later become the model for the WEA National Standard Program.

    b.   In 1977, Paul Petzoldt and a group of college professors discussed the need for college-level professional training programs for the development of wilderness leaders and educators. On October 22, 1977, the Wilderness Use Education Association (WUEA) was created.

    c.   In 1978, WUEA was incorporated as a non-profit organization in the state of Wyoming. In 1980, it was officially renamed WEA and Paul Petzoldt was appointed as Executive Director.

    d.   **Wilderness Education Association philosophy**
Through the processing and evaluation of leadership experiences, the WEA prepares individuals to lead safe, enjoyable, and environmentally sound backcountry outings. The WEA provides leadership training through a decentralized network of colleges, universities, and outdoor programs which emphasize the development of quality decision making and sound judgment.

    e.   WEA courses typically consist of students who are seeking professional outdoor leadership development.

B.   **A Brief Chronology of WEA History**
    1976 - Dr. Frank Lupton and Paul Petzoldt met together and decided to include a wilderness backpacking expedition in Wyoming as part of the curriculum of a "Camping and Outdoor Education" course taught by Dr. Lupton in the Department of Recreation, Park Administration & Tourism at Western Illinois University. The success of the experience prompted experimentation with similar programs throughout the summer of 1977.

1977 - Dr. Frank Lupton, Paul Petzoldt, Dr. Robert Christie (then Director of Bradford Woods at Indiana University), and Charles Gregory (then Director of Stone Valley Outdoor Education Center at Pennsylvania State University) met together on October 22, 1977 to discuss the need to create a wilderness leadership certification program which could gain national acceptance. This meeting ended with the formation of the Wilderness Use Education Association (later to become the Wilderness Education Association). The participants agreed that national certifying programs needed to be established at three levels:
  • **User certification** - certifying skills competency for wilderness travel
  • **Leadership certification** - certifying competency to lead others into wilderness areas
  • **Instructor certification** - certifying competency to prepare leaders who have the skills and leadership qualities necessary for wilderness travel

1977 - Experimental fall, summer, and winter WUEA courses were initiated by several colleges and universities throughout the country, and also through WUEA headquarters at the Paul Petzoldt Lodge in Driggs, Idaho.

1978 - An advisory committee of professionals from all over the U.S. was formed to provide input and suggestions for improvement of WUEA programs.

1978 - WUEA was incorporated in the state of Wyoming as a non-profit organization.

1980 - WUEA was officially renamed the Wilderness Education Association (WEA).
  • Paul Petzoldt was appointed as Executive Director of WEA.

1984 - Sandra Braun became the second WEA Executive Director. This period saw a major expansion of programs, some offered by WEA affiliates and some sponsored by the central WEA office in Driggs, Idaho. A major debate evolved over WEA's future:
  • WEA programs at the home office were perceived by some as siphoning students away from university affiliate programs.

- The financial resources of the central organization remained inadequate to effectively service and monitor the quality of affiliate courses.

1986 - WEA headquarters was temporarily moved to Western Illinois University.
- WEA Board of Trustees decided that all home office courses must be eliminated in order to gain national recognition as an accrediting body for outdoor leadership training programs. From this time forward, courses would only be run through affiliates.

1987 - WEA headquarters was moved to North Country Community College in Saranac Lake, NY as a result of a grant provided by the Adirondack North Country Association. The organization became more focused on building an affiliate network and membership base, and on providing professional services for its membership.

1988 - Mark Wagstaff was hired as Executive Director. WEA experienced significant growth as reflected in affiliate membership which rose from 6 to 30 between 1988 and 1992.

C. **WEA Mission Statement and Approach**
1. **WEA Mission Statement**
    The purpose of the Wilderness Education Association is to promote the professionalization of outdoor leadership and to thereby improve the safety and quality of outdoor trips and enhance the conservation of the wild outdoors.
2. **The WEA Approach**
    a. WEA certifies outdoor leaders through programs offered in affiliation with colleges, universities, and outdoor programs.
    b. WEA depends on its membership for funding to develop programs and fulfill its mission. In return, WEA provides its membership with a variety of benefits and services.
    c. WEA continues to review its curriculum and develop new programs to serve the needs of the profession.

d. WEA provides consulting services to affiliates and other outdoor organizations.

    e. WEA provides support for organizations and individuals doing research in the wilderness education field.

D. **WEA 18-Point Curriculum**

The purpose of this section is to ensure that participants recognize the existence of the formal WEA curriculum from which the course content is taught.

Judgment

Good judgment is the umbrella that covers the 18 points. It is the pervasive leadership quality that grows from the exercise of decision making in a leadership role. The development of good judgment is the philosophical and educational objective underlying all 18 points.

1. Decision Making and Problem Solving
2. Leadership
3. Expedition Behavior and Group Dynamics
4. Environmental Ethics
5. Basic Camping Skills
6. Nutrition and Rations Planning
7. Equipment and Clothing Selection and Use
8. Weather
9. Health and Sanitation
10. Travel Techniques
11. Navigation
12. Safety and Risk Management
13. Wilderness Emergency Procedures and Treatment
14. Natural and Cultural History
15. Specialized Travel/Adventure Activity
16. Communication Skills
17. Trip Planning
18. Teaching, Processing, and Transference

E. **WEA Certification**

1. **Wilderness Steward, certificate of participation**
The Wilderness Steward Program was developed in the late 1980s and is still in a stage of growth and experimentation. Many Stewardship Courses are modeled after the shakedown portion of a WEA National Standard Program and expose participants to one or more areas of the 18-point curriculum.

(The shakedown is a short trip at the beginning of a WEA course designed to provide an intense philosophical orientation and skills preparation for the remaining time in the field). A certificate of participation is granted to an individual who completes a Wilderness Steward Program.

2. **Certified Outdoor Leader**
   a. This is granted to an individual who successfully completes a National Standard Program. This certifies that an individual is able to:
      (1) Teach others how to use and enjoy the wilderness with minimum impact
      (2) Safely lead others in the wild outdoors
      (3) Exercise good judgment and leadership and fully recognize his or her leadership abilities and limitations
      (4) Demonstrate a basic standard of outdoor knowledge and experience based on the WEA 18-point curriculum
   b. Certification records are maintained and stored at the WEA national office. With the student's permission, these records are available to prospective employers. Certification records are evaluation documents of a student's performance.

3. **Certification apprentice instructor**
   An apprentice assumes head instructor duties while on an NSP under the direct supervision of a head instructor who provides performance feedback throughout the course. Although apprentice instructors do not receive a certification, it is a step towards attaining instructor certification.

4. **Certification instructor**
   A certification instructor plans, leads, teaches, and evaluates a National Standard Program. In order to be certified as an instructor, candidates usually apprentice on at least one course. Instructors may be certified in one of the following ways:
   a. They may be recommended for instructor status by a head instructor with whom they apprentice.
   b. They may successfully complete an instructor's course.

5. **The WEA and its affiliates**
   a. **National Standard Program affiliates**
      The WEA accredits colleges, universities, and select outdoor programs to offer the National Standard Program.
   b. The WEA NSP affiliate relationship is based upon the following:
      (1) The affiliate submits a written proposal to the Board of Trustees for approval.
      (2) The affiliate will teach the 18-point curriculum.
      (3) The affiliate will use the WEA standard evaluation and certification procedures.
      (4) The affiliate will pay an annual accreditation fee and a per-student certification fee.
      (5) A certified WEA instructor will teach the course.
   c. **Steward Program affiliates**
      The WEA recognizes colleges, universities, and select programs to offer the Steward Program.
   d. The WEA Steward affiliate relationship is based upon the following:
      (1) The affiliate submits a written proposal to the WEA office, where the executive director and a Steward committee will review it for approval.
      (2) The affiliate will teach one or more components of the 18-point curriculum.
      (3) The affiliate will pay an annual fee and a per-student fee.
      (4) A certified WEA leader or instructor will teach the course.
   e. **Benefits of the affiliation system**
      (1) Affiliates gain an established college-level curriculum which is constantly reviewed.
      (2) The WEA is free to focus on curriculum development and educational support.
      (3) WEA accreditation benefits students with increased credibility and competitiveness in the job market.

(4) All NSP and Steward participants receive a one-year membership in the WEA with all associated benefits. These benefits include:
   (a) Job referral service
   (b) Discounts on equipment purchases
   (c) Discounts on wilderness medical training
   (d) Discounts on registration for the WEA national conference
   (e) Discounts on outdoor publications

6. **Current affiliates**
   This would be an appropriate time for the instructor to review the current affiliates.

IV. INSTRUCTIONAL STRATEGIES & MATERIALS:
   A. **Timing**
   This topic is usually taught as time permits. It is particularly suitable for a rainy day or a rest day.

   B. **Strategies**
   1. **Lecture**
   This approach is most appropriate when participants have little or no knowledge of the topic (see "Teaching Techniques" lesson for different teaching strategies).

   2. **The "WEA Minute"**
   Using the WEA chronology of events, students are asked to volunteer to prepare a short presentation (1-3 minutes) based on the lesson content. Each day a presentation is given at the daily debriefing or at some other appropriate time.

   3. **Student-led presentations**
   Students are asked to take a portion of the lesson content and present it to the group. Students should be encouraged to use their creativity to make the presentations as interesting as possible (i.e., impersonations, skits, etc.).

   4. **Storytelling**
   If a staff or group member has personal knowledge of the evolution of WEA, their personal experiences could be used as a basis for a storytelling/discussion approach to the topic. A campfire or other teachable moment may provide a good opportunity for this approach.

181

C. **Activities**

The instructor can provide participants with an example of a common outdoor activity that reflects the different philosophy of each organization. It should be pointed out that the differences are sometimes subtle, and an observer may find the distinctions among the programs blurred depending on the instructor, location, and/or situation. The following is an example:

Map & compass activity

1. **Outward Bound**: The group is asked to travel from point A to point B. Participants are given minimal instruction in map and compass use. The focus of the exercise is to build group unity and individual confidence as group members work together to reach the objective. Participants debrief the experience in terms of their personal growth and group dynamics.

2. **National Outdoor Leadership School**: The group is asked to travel from point A to point B. Participants are given extensive formal instruction in map and compass use including the rationale behind the techniques used. The focus of the exercise is to teach specific map and compass skills. Debriefing and journaling of the activity may or may not occur.

3. **Wilderness Education Association**: The group is asked to travel from point A to point B. Participants are given extensive formal instruction in map and compass use including the rationale behind the techniques used. The focus of the exercise is to provide decision-making opportunities and teach specific map and compass skills. Participants debrief the experience in terms of the leadership and decision-making skills related to the activity as well as what they learned about navigation. Students are required to reflect on their experience through journaling.

25. Weather

by Michael Kudish Ph.D.

I. **GOAL**: To have participants predict weather in the field as accurately as possible using a compass, a barometer, and their senses.

II. **OBJECTIVES**:
   A. Participants will be able to explain why weather is difficult to predict accurately.
   B. Participants will be able to use a barometer or altimeter to predict weather.
   C. Participants will be able to identify wind direction and use it to predict weather.
   D. Participants will be able to use different cloud formations in helping to predict weather.

III. **CONTENT**:
   A. **Weather is difficult to accurately predict**
      1. Atmospheric movements are mostly random in nature.
      2. No two weather systems, masses, or fronts are alike.
      3. Weather observers and weather stations are too far apart to get an accurate reading of regional weather.
      4. Some weather phenomena are very localized (e.g., showers and flurries).

   B. **Barometric Pressure**
      1. Barometric pressure is the pressure created by the weight of air above us.
         a. Because the molecules are further apart, warm air is less dense than cold and holds more moisture.
         b. Warm air rises, cold air sinks.

2.   As air cools and sinks, it becomes more dense and causes higher pressure. This denser air keeps other systems away, therefore skies in a high pressure system remain clear.

3.   Air in a low pressure system is less dense than in a high, which causes it to draw winds (which are often moist) into the system. Therefore, low pressure systems often bring cloudy, stormy weather.

C.   **Barometer/Altimeter**

1.   **A barometer or altimeter can be used to measure elevations**
       Barometers or altimeters are affected by elevation changes. Pressure drops about 1 in. (actually 1.05 in. to 1.10 in./2.66 cm. to 2.79 cm.) or 25.4 mm., 33.86 mb. (millibars) of mercury for each 1000 ft./305 m. of elevation gained.

2.   **A barometer or altimeter can be used to predict weather**

       a.   The following guidelines are usually dependable although exceptions occur:

              (1)   **Steady or nil change in pressure:** more of the same weather and often not windy.

              (2)   **Rising pressure:** clearing but watch for instability which may mean showers in the mountains.

              (3)   **Falling pressure:** clouding over and precipitation may follow unless the storm passes over far enough away.

              (4)   **Rapid change, up or down:** a rapid change in the weather, usually windy.

       b.   The average pressure adjusted to sea level is 30.00 in. (762 mm., 1016 mb.). Always adjust the barometer to sea level readings. Set the barometer at home (from a weather report) and know what the elevations in the field will be so the barometer can be reset before leaving for field trips. (See Figure 25-1.)

              (1)   **Pressure of 30.60 in. (777 mm., 1036 mb.) in winter and steady, dry, clear, nil wind:** coldest nights, sometimes ground fog in the morning.

(2) **Pressure of 30.25 in. (768 mm., 1024 mb.) or more during the rest of the year:** coldest nights, frosts in spring and fall, sometimes ground fog in the morning.

(3) **Pressure of 29.00 in. (737 mm., 982 mb.) in severe winter or early spring storms, or in hurricanes:** rain or snow, windy.

(4) **Pressure of 29.75 in. (756 mm., 1007 mb.) or lower:** rain or snow, windy.

(5) **General rule:**
  (a) **High pressure**
    Summer = clear weather
    Winter = clear and cold weather
  (b) **Low pressure**
    Summer = rainy, stormy weather
    Winter = rain or snow

IN	MM	MB
31.00	787	1050
30.00	762	1016
29.92	760	1013
29.53	750	1000
29.00	737	982
28.00	711	948
27.00	686	914

1 IN = 25.4 MM = 33.86 MB
1 MM = 1.333 MB

Figure 25 -1 Barometer Scales Compared

D. **Wind**

It is virtually impossible for the weather to change without wind. It is the wind, at varying elevations, that blows in different weather. The following guidelines are an example of how weather is affected by wind in the northeastern United States:

1. **South or southwest air from the south Atlantic Ocean or Gulf of Mexico:** above normal temperatures, humid, poor visibility, warm nights, frequent showers, partly cloudy in between showers. When south or southwest winds strengthen, a cold front may be approaching.

2. **North or northwest:** cooler, drier air from Canadian interior, colder than normal temperatures, instability, flurries, and showers. Most severe from November through January.

3. **West:** usually fair with normal temperatures.

4. **Southeast, east, or northeast:** coastal storm approaching, rain or snow if a storm is close enough, wind normally shifts to northwest after the storm.

5. **North to northeast:** Canadian maritime air, cold, cloudy, and wet (but rare).

6. **No wind, high pressure at center of air mass:** fair, warm days and cold nights with low humidity.

E. **Temperature changes with change in elevation**

Temperature changes can be used as a guide to determine changes in barometric pressure. If the temperature changes (over at least several hours) more than the degrees given below for every 1000 ft. (305 m.) of elevation gained or lost, then this would indicate that the barometric pressure is changing.

1. 3° F (6° C) per 1000 ft. (305 m.) of ascent is average

2. 2° F (4° C) per 1000 ft. (305 m.) of ascent when wet and/or windy indicates a low pressure system

3. 4° F (8° C) per 1000 ft. (305 m.) of ascent when dry and/or calm indicates a high pressure system

4. 5° F (11° C) per 1000 ft. (305 m.) of ascent is the theoretical maximum possible, with 0% relative humidity and absolutely still air, rarely realized in nature.

F. **Clouds**
   1. **Types of clouds**
      The types of clouds are classified according to how
      they are formed in the atmosphere.
      a. **Cumulus**
         (1) These are formed by rising air currents at
             almost any altitude.
         (2) These are the classic, puffy, white clouds.
         (3) These appear in the middle of a high
             pressure air mass, mainly building up in
             the afternoon. Clouds with flat bottoms
             above mountains indicate fair weather.
      b. **Stratus** (*stratus* refers to the word *layer*).
         These sheets or horizontal layers are formed
         when air cools to the dew point (the point at
         which air becomes saturated and reaches 100%
         humidity).
   2. **Families of clouds**
      Families of clouds are classified according to their
      altitude.
      a. **High:** these are 20,000-25,000 ft. above the earth
         and consist of ice crystals.
         Types of high clouds
         (1) **Cirrus** (*cirrus* refers to the word *streak*): thin,
             wispy, and delicate. These don't contain
             precipitation but may indicate
             precipitation within the next 24 hours.
             These so-called "mares' tails" (scattered
             and wispy) often consist of ice crystals and
             often indicate approaching precipitation.
         (2) **Cirrocumulus:** rippled and thin. These
             often consist of ice crystals that reflect light
             and create a "halo" around the sun or
             moon. These are also known as a
             "mackerel sky." They often indicate fair
             weather but may also bring brief showers.
      b. **Middle:** these are about 10,000 ft. to 6,500 ft.
         above the earth , but are sometimes as high as
         20,000 ft. They consist of water and may
         contain some ice crystals.

Types of middle clouds
(1) **Altocumulus** (*alto* refers to the middle range): puffy, white, or gray. These indicate fair weather with precipitation likely within 8-10 hours.
(2) **Altostratus:** gray or blue. These usually bring light rain or snow.

c. **Low:** these are about 6,500 ft. or less above the earth.

Types of low clouds
(1) **Stratus:** low, uniform, and thin. They consist of water droplets and may produce a fine drizzle but not a rain.
(2) **Nimbostratus:** low, thick, and dark gray. These yield steady rain or snow.
(3) **Stratocumulus:** thick, gray, and irregular. These don't produce precipitation but often change into nimbostratus.

d. **Towering:** these range from low altitudes up to 40,000 ft.
Cumulonimbus: cauliflower-shaped with flat, anvil-like tops. These are classic thunderheads and produce heavy thunderstorms, rain, snow, or hail.

3. **Red sunrises and sunsets**
a. A red sunset indicates that tomorrow's weather may be dry. Dry air refracts red light. This indicates that clear dry air is to the west, which is often the direction from which storms come.
b. Red sunrises are caused by reflections in moist air that may indicate rain later in the day.
c. Thus there is some truth to the saying "red sky at morning, sailors take warning. Red sky at night, sailor's delight."

4. **Ground fog and/or dew**
a. **Fog**
(1) Morning fog is the result of moisture in damp air that condenses in the cold of the night and is usually burned off by the heat of the morning sun.
(2) Late afternoon or evening fog is usually formed as moisture falls through warmer air and often indicates a coming storm.

b. **Dew**
   (1) Since warm air holds more moisture than cold air, as air cools its relative humidity increases until the moisture in it reaches the maximum that it can hold at that temperature (this is called the dew point). If the air continues to cool, some moisture in it has to condense and may be deposited as dew.
   (2) At night, the air near the surface of the earth cools. If it cools below its dew point, dew forms on the ground.
   (3) Dew is most common on calm, cloudless, cool nights. Since both wind and clouds reduce the cooling rate of air near the surface of the earth, temperatures drop more slowly and the air may not reach its dew point before the sun rises again in the morning.
   (4) No dew at night may indicate rain by morning. No dew in the morning may indicate rain by the next day.

G. **Other factors to consider when forecasting weather**
   1. Season
   2. Local conditions (e.g., mountains, large lakes, frost pockets, aspect, elevation, microclimate)
      a. **Mountain and valley winds**
         Since wind (moving air) takes the path of least resistance, winds can be quite strong in lower elevations such as valleys and mountain passes. As the wind "squeezes" through these narrow areas, it picks up speed.
      b. **Deserts**
         As very hot air quickly rises, surrounding air will rush in and fill the void, creating "heat lows" such as dust devils.
   3. Since many animals are particularly sensitive to changes in atmospheric pressure, they often give signs that indicate weather changes (e.g., before a storm, some birds such as woodpeckers and blue jays are often very noisy, but insects will stop making noise).

4. Average weather conditions and historical weather patterns for the area can be obtained from National Weather Service publications. The following agencies publish weather statistics and can provide climatological summaries of regional weather.
    a. National Oceanic and Atmospheric Administration (NOAA) Weather Radio, National Climatic Center, Federal Building, Asheville, NC, 28801
    b. National Oceanographic and Atmospheric Association, Rockville, MD, 20852

IV. **INSTRUCTIONAL STRATEGIES & MATERIALS:**
A. **Timing**
    This lesson is effectively taught using "teachable moments" when changes in weather occur.

B. **Strategies**
    1. Participants can choose a "weatherperson" to record temperature highs and lows and weather patterns during the course. These patterns can be studied to better understand weather systems.
    2. This is a good lesson for students who have a special interest in meteorology to instruct.

C. **Materials**
    1. Barometer(s)
    2. Compass(es)

26. Food Identification

I. **GOAL:** To have participants identify food items and gain a
    basic knowledge of food preparation considerations.

II. **OBJECTIVES:**
    A. Participants will understand the WEA rationing philosophy.
    B. Participants will understand why the food is packaged
        the way it is.
    C. Participants will be able to care for the food selected.
    D. Participants will be able to identify food items.
    E. Participants will be aware of cooking tips for specific
        food items.

III. **CONTENT:**
    A. **Total Food Planning**
        This process is based on determining caloric needs and
        making sure you have enough food to meet those caloric
        needs with as little weight as possible. (See "Nutrition
        and Rations Planning" lesson for more on this topic.) The
        advantages of total food planning are:
        1. A large variety of foods can be used to provide for
            an endless variety of meals.
        2. It allows spontaneity and creativity in cooking and
            eating.
        3. It does away with the need to plan specific meals.
            Individuals can eat what they want, when they
            want, and meet caloric needs.
        4. The financial savings are generally substantial by
            minimizing pre-packaged meals and cooking from
            scratch.

© 1992
The Wilderness Education Association
P.O. Box 89
Saranac Lake, New York 12983
(518) 891-2915 ext. 254

B. **Food Packaging — Why Plastic Containers, Plastic Bags, and Overhand Knots?**
  1. **Plastic containers and plastic bags**
     a. They are lightweight compared to glass, tin cans, and aluminum foil.
     b. They are safer than glass (because glass breaks).
     c. They are easy to pack and carry out.
     d. They are lightweight and can be easily carried out.
     e. Some plastic containers (e.g. film canisters for spices) are reusable and therefore good "environmental" choices.
  2. **Overhand knots instead of twist ties**
     a. Twist ties can puncture holes in other bags.
     b. Twist ties can be easily lost, creating litter.
     c. Zippered plastic bags are useful for short trips only; "zippers" become plugged with food and function poorly.
  3. **Wrapping cheese**
     In hot and humid weather it is sometimes advisable to wrap cheese in freezer wrap or cheese cloth. This helps absorb oils and will delay mold.

C. **Food Care and Organization**
  1. **Organizing food bags**
     a. Organize foods alphabetically, by meals, by color, or any other preferred method.
     b. Once foods are categorized, keep them organized by returning them to their same food bags so they can be found next time they are needed.
  2. **Keeping food bags clean**
     a. If bags break, rebag them and clean up as soon as possible.
     b. As garbage accumulates, keep it in one plastic bag.
  3. **Plastic bags**
     a. Keep the knots loose. If knots get tight, twist the working end and push it back through the knot to untie it.
     b. Lift the bags from below the knot or from the bottom of the bag (so knots don't tighten).
     c. Double bag food items that would suffer disastrous consequences if they leak or puncture (i.e. spaghetti and flour).

4. **Plastic containers**
   a. They may not be leak proof; if in doubt, store them in plastic bags. Messy or sticky items such as honey should be bagged to prevent soiling other items in the food bag.
   b. Handle containers with care — wide-mouthed container lids sometimes crack.
5. **Food preservation**
   The food chosen for a trip should not spoil. However, in hotter portions of the country, care should be taken to keep items such as cheese, margarine, and meats cool by keeping them in the shade. This will:
   • provide easier handling
   • prevent mold growth
   • prevent deterioration of taste (although nutritional quality remains the same).

D. **Food Identification**
   1. *Go through the food bags identifying each food item and giving preparation ideas. (See Appendix at the end of this chapter for food list.)*
   2. **General food preparation ideas**
      a. Fruits, vegetables, and TVP should be rehydrated in hot water before adding to the meal.
      b. Flour makes a good thickener. A good white sauce can be made with flour, water, margarine, salt, pepper, and other spices of choice.
      c. Vegetable oil, margarine, and powdered milk should be added to most dinners for the nutritional gain.

IV. **INSTRUCTIONAL STRATEGIES & MATERIALS:**
   A. **Timing**
      1. This unit is designed to help students through the maze of plastic bags, identifying and getting general ideas on how to prepare food.
      2. It is best taught on the second or third day in a relaxed setting.
      3. It can be prefaced with an "Introductory Cooking" class so students can cook their first meals. (WEA affiliate North Country Community College teaches "Granola Preparation" the first morning in the field and "Food Identification" the second or third day.)

4. This class may be followed with specific classes on "Introductory Cooking," "Frying and Baking" (both baking powder and yeast), and "Nutrition and Rations Planning." Cooking techniques are also taught on an individual basis using teachable moments. Regardless of how the topic is taught, it is important to encourage creativity and experimentation. Have a *NOLS Cookery* or similar publication available for participants to use for ideas.

B. **Strategies**
  1. As the instructor identifies each item, participants can identify food from their own bags. This allows participants to become aware of all items they have brought.
  2. A list of suggested food items and preparation tips has been provided as an appendix to this lesson plan.

C. **Activities**
  Identification of food can be done in any combination of the following ways:
  1. Pull foods out randomly and pass them around. Comment on how to identify them and provide preparation ideas.
  2. Sort foods by similar color and point out the subtle differences between foods.
  3. Go through foods by meal groups — dinners, breakfasts, and lunches.
  4. Go through a "Master Food List" alphabetically. (See appendix of "Nutrition and Rations Planning" lesson for a "Master Food List.")

D. **Materials**
  1. All food bags
  2. *NOLS Cookery* or similar publication

Appendix: Suggested Food Items and Preparation Tips

Apples (dried): Add to hot cereal, eat raw, or rehydrate for baking.
Apricots (dried): Add to hot cereal, eat raw, or rehydrate for baking.
Baking Powder
Beef Base: Start with less than a teaspoon as it is very salty. Add base to water.
Brownie Mix: Mix:water = 8:1.
Bulgar: Prepare the same way as rice. Can be used with or instead of rice, or combined with veggies to make a tabouli salad.
Candy
Cashews
Cheese Cake Mix: Add to already-mixed milk, stir, and let set. Mix:milk = 1:1.
Cheese: Cheddar, Mozzarella, Muenster, Colby.
Chicken Base: Start with less than a teaspoon as it is very salty. Add base to water.
Chili base: Mix with water to taste.
Cocoa: Mix with water and/or milk.
Coconut: Add to granola or use for baking.
Cornmeal: Add to pancake mix, breads, tortillas, etc.
Cream of Wheat: Water:Cream of wheat = 4:1.
Dates: Add to hot cereal, eat raw, or rehydrate for baking.
Egg Noodles: Bring water to a boil, then add noodles and about a tablespoon of oil (to keep noodles from sticking together).
Fruit Drink: Orange, Lemon, Fruit
Flour (unbleached and whole wheat): Whole wheat can be mixed with unbleached flour. Use between a 2:1 and 1:1 ratio (unbleached : whole wheat).
Gingerbread Mix: Add enough water to form a thick, runny consistency.
Honey: Use in addition to or instead of other sweeteners.
Jello: Use as a high energy hot drink. (It is difficult to make Jello gel in the field.)
Macaroni: Bring water to a boil, then add noodles and about a tablespoon of oil (to keep pasta from sticking together).
Magarine: Add a little to every dinner for a good source of energy.
Milk (powdered): Mixes best when cold. Water:milk = 2:1.
Mushroom Soup Base: Add water to base, to taste.
Nuts (mixed)
Oatmeal (rolled, not instant): Cooks in 10-12 minutes. Water:oatmeal = 2:1.
Onions (dried): Rehydrate 12-15 minutes in hot water.

Pancake Mix: Add water.

Peanut Butter

Peanuts

Pepperoni: Can be cut up in dinners, or used for lunch.

Pepper (dried): Rehydrate 12-15 minutes in hot water.

Popcorn

Potatoes (sliced): Rehydrate by covering with water in a fry pan. Let sit for 10 -15 minutes (don't stir or turn over).

Potatoes (powdered): Good as a thickener, in potato pancakes, or just as potatoes.

Prunes: Add to hot cereal, eat raw, or rehydrate for baking.

Pudding (instant chocolate or vanilla): Add milk, stir, and let set. Milk : pudding = 4:1.

Raisins (regular and golden): Add to hot cereal, eat raw, or rehydrate for baking.

Rice: Add to water, then boil for 15-20 minutes. Water:rice = 2:1.

Salt

Soy Sauce

Spaghetti: Bring water to a boil, then add pasta and about a tablespoon of oil (to keep pasta from sticking together).

Sugar (white and brown): Use in addition to or instead of other sweetener.

Sunflower seeds

Tea (regular and spiced)

Tomato base: Add water to base.

Trail mix

TVP: An inexpensive meat substitute. It has meat texture but very little taste and no fat. Best if rehydrated in hot water for 15-20 minutes.

Vanilla

Vegetables (dried, mixed): Rehydrate 12-15 minutes in hot water.

Vegetable oil: Add to dinners, use for popcorn, pancakes, etc.

Vinegar

Walnuts

Wheatena: Water:Wheatena = 4:1.

Yeast

27. Food Protection

I. **GOAL**: To have participants properly protect food rations from animals under a variety of circumstances.

II. **OBJECTIVES**:
A. Participants will be able to explain the need for food protection.
B. Participants will be able to describe the general principles of food protection.
C. Participants will be able to demonstrate two different systems of food protection.

III. **CONTENT**:
A. **The Need for Food Protection**
1. **The consequences of animals accessing food should be obvious**
a. Campers may lose some or all of their food.
b. Food bags and other equipment may be damaged or destroyed.
c. In some areas there is a potential for campers to be injured, or in rare cases even killed, from animals coming into camp in search of food.
2. **Types of animals searching for food bags**
a. Insects
b. Mice: particularly common in heavily camped areas.
c. Chipmunks
d. Squirrels: squirrels can readily chew through nylon and run up, down, or across nearly any hanging line, and are considered by many to be the most ruthless animal encountered in the outdoors.
e. Raccoons: creative, intelligent, and dexterous.
f. Bears: creative, intelligent, inquisitive, and potentially dangerous.

© 1992
The Wilderness Education Association
P.O. Box 89
Saranac Lake, New York 12983
(518) 891-2915 ext. 254

3. **Ethical considerations**
   Although it might be cute to feed chipmunks or other critters, it is detrimental to them.
   a. It may cause wildlife to lose their fear of humans and create a dependence which could cause them to starve once people leave. When humans supply food for animals, the animals risks losing their food-finding skills because they stop using them.
   b. Attracting animals may cause additional risks, such as safety problems for both the animals and people (e.g., rabid animals, bears), and sanitation problems (e.g., eating from a pot that a raccoon has licked).
   c. Even the slightest trace of human food alters the ecosystem.
   d. A bear that is habituated to eating trail food is essentially a dead bear. Bears that are trapped and relocated have a very low rate of survival. Therefore, if a bear gets *your* trail food, *you* are responsible for its death!

B. **General Principles of Food Protection**
   1. **Determine whether it is necessary to hang bags**
      It is a general policy at WEA affiliate North Country Community College to protect food bags in the Adirondack Park.
      a. Hang bags each night, except when camping in the most remote areas where animals have not learned of our existence.
      b. Hang bags when the group is in an area where bears are known to have invaded camps.
   2. **Look for a site to hang food bags during daylight hours**
   3. **Find a site which meets the following requirements**
      a. For small mammals, it should be at least four feet (1 m.) off the ground and four feet from the nearest tree.
      b. For bears, it should be at least 12 feet (3.5 m.) off the ground and six feet (2 m.) from the nearest tree.

4. **Select a method which will work best for the site found**
   a. **Two-tree method**: ideal and most secure method (Figure 27-1).
   b. **Single-tree method**: works well in many instances, particularly for protection from small mammals (Figure 27-2).
   c. **Single-branch method**: works best with a lightweight food bag and a strong branch (Figure 27-3).

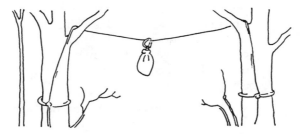

Figure 27-1   Two-tree Method

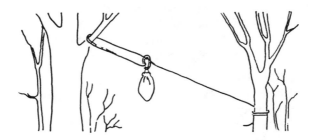

Figure 27-2   Single-tree Method

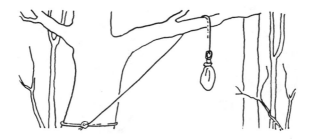

Figure 27-3   Single-branch Method

IV. INSTRUCTIONAL STRATEGIES & MATERIALS:

A. Timing

This class can be taught using the teachable moment at the beginning of a course and before problems develop. Depending on the types of animals in the region, it can be followed up with a more formal class as time permits or circumstances demand.

B. Strategies

1. This class lends itself nicely to student instruction. It is a relatively simple class, yet provides an opportunity for the demonstration of many elements essential to good teaching.
2. Many instructors use a lecture/demonstration approach followed by student practice of the skill.
3. For grizzly bear country or country where black bears present a problem:

   a. Bears have an acute sense of smell and may be attracted to the smell of food or any other odor (except human scent).
   b. Hang food and other smellables such as soaps, toothpaste, lip balm, sunscreen, toothbrushes, insect repellant, unused film cartridges, and first aid kits.
   c. Hang food and smellables during the day if the group leaves camp.

C. Materials

1. Rope: at least 40 feet (12 m.) of 1/4" (.5 cm.) diameter nylon cord
2. Carabiner: 1 or 2 (optional)
3. Small pulley (optional)
4. Food bags

28. Food Waste Disposal

I. **GOAL**: To have participants dispose of food waste in a variety of appropriate ways and understand which method to use in a given situation.

II. **OBJECTIVES**:
A. Participants will understand the importance of proper food waste disposal.
B. Participants will be able to use a fire for disposal of food waste.
C. Participants will understand the option of packing food back to "civilization" and disposing of it appropriately.
D. Participants will understand the importance of cooking no more food than can be eaten.
E. Participants will understand why and when each means of food disposal is appropriate.

III. **CONTENT**:
A. **Why show concern in how we dispose of food waste?**
1. To prevent contamination of the water supply.
    a. Eutrophication (see "Bathing and Washing" lesson).
    b. Aesthetics: who wants to see food waste on the bottom of the lake?
    c. Illegal: It is illegal to randomly dispose of waste in virtually all federal and state wilderness areas.
2. To minimize alteration of wildlife feeding and migration habits.
3. To minimize wildlife (e.g., squirrel, chipmunk, raccoon, bear, insects) feeding on human food waste.
4. To minimize negative impact on the aesthetics of a campsite and cooking area.
5. To increase the social carrying capacity of the wilderness area.

© 1992
The Wilderness Education Association
P.O. Box 89
Saranac Lake, New York 12983
(518) 891-2915 ext. 254

B. **Disposal of Waste Water and Food Particles**
 1. The utmost care should be taken to eliminate all food particles from waste water. This can be accomplished by straining waste water through a wire or nylon screen. Food particles should be bagged and packed out or completely burned off in a hot fire.
 2. In the absence of a screen, a makeshift strainer can be constructed. Pack some forest litter inside a plastic bag and puncture holes in the bottom of the bag.
 3. Unless the water has been carefully screened first, sump holes are discouraged as a waste water disposal practice. Field experience indicates that these holes are frequently dug up by animals, creating aesthetic problems as well as encouraging animals to alter their normal feeding habits.

C. **Fires for Food Waste Disposal**
 1. Dig a shallow hole in one corner of the firepit (or fireplace) and pour food waste into the hole.
    a. For this to be effective, the solid waste must be burned or animals will dig up the firepit later. Strain the liquid waste into the shallow hole and place solid waste directly into the fire.
    b. Pour solid food waste into a firepit only if there is a fire burning. Otherwise, waste may not get burned and it is likely that animals will dig up the pit later.
    c. Leftover solid food waste should be removed from the firepit and disposed of using an alternative method before the duff is replaced or before camp is broken. This minimizes the risk that animals will dig up the firepit later.

D. **Broadcasting Food Outside the Campsite**
 1. During extended expeditions in pristine or "virgin" campsites (one where there is no evidence of previous use), food can be taken to the edge of the campsite area and strewn about. The use of this practice is subject to considerable debate. Good judgment is necessary in deciding whether this practice is acceptable in any given situation.

2. Considerations when broadcasting food outside of camp:
   a. Broadcasting should not be employed in designated or heavily camped areas because of its tendency to disrupt animal behavior.
   b. Spread the food out evenly, so that unsightly clumps of food are not left.
   c. This practice is not advisable in bear country.

E. **Packing Food Out**
   1. If in doubt, pack food out.
   2. Try not to cook more food than you can eat and minimize the amount of food waste that must be packed out.

IV. **INSTRUCTIONAL STRATEGIES & MATERIALS:**
   A. **Timing**
      This information can be taught using the teachable moment within the first few days of the course.

   B. **Strategies**
      1. In grizzly bear country or country where black bears present a problem:
         a. Burn garbage and uneaten food or hang it in a bear bag.
         b. Put wet garbage and uneaten food in plastic bags and hang them in a bear bag.
         c. Use a sump to dispose of dirty dishwater and cooking liquids.

   C. **Activities**
      1. As the group enters a campsite, ask participants what type of food disposal might be most appropriate and why.
      2. Depending on the age level and motivation, instructors may have to monitor the group closely to insure compliance with proper food disposal techniques.

   D. **Materials**
      1. Shovel
      2. Firepit or fireplace
      3. Food waste
      4. Wire or nylon screen
      5. "Natural" screen of litter in a perforated plastic bag

29. Frying and Baking

I.   **GOAL**: Participants will be able to prepare and bake a variety of foods suitable for consumption in the backcountry.

II. **OBJECTIVES**:
   A. Participants will be able to discuss some reasons for baking while on a wilderness expedition.
   B. Participants will demonstrate an ability to properly use the major tools and utensils employed in baking, including fry-pan ovens and stove-top ovens/ring pans.
   C. Participants will demonstrate an ability to build a fire and oven platform suitable for baking.
   D. Participants will be able to describe the basic recipe for "bannock" and several simple alternatives.
   E. Participants will successfully bake edible foods on both a fire and a stove.

III. **CONTENT:**
   A. **The Joys of Baking**
       Preparing nutritious, tasty, baked goods can directly contribute to the success of any backcountry expedition.
       1. **Baking and the diet**
           a. Baked goods help add variety to the common backcountry menu. Biscuits, buns, and bread all greatly enhance the sense of creativity associated with good cooking.
           b. Baked goods can add courses to a meal which otherwise would be missing (e.g., appetizers, desserts, etc.).
           c. Baked goods provide a source of protein and carbohydrates.
       2. **Baking and group morale/expedition behavior**
           a. Sharing baked goods at the end of a tough day can renew group enthusiasm and spirit.

© 1992
The Wilderness Education Association
P.O. Box 89
Saranac Lake, New York 12983
(518) 891-2915 ext. 254

b.   Baking allows individuals in the group to
demonstrate skills and creativity in a non-
competitive way.

c.   Baking for the group and sharing with others
can serve as a means of showing affection and
caring. "Nothin' says lovin' like somethin' from
the oven."

d.   Baking in small groups provides an opportunity for group members to share a relaxing,
productive, social occasion that fosters communication, mutual cooperation, and understanding.

B.   **The Tools**
1.   **Basic cooking utensils** (see "Granola Preparation"
lesson).

2.   **The fry-pan oven**
a.   The fry-pan oven is usually a teflon-coated 10"
fry pan and an aluminum 10" lid.

b.   The fry-pan oven is designed to bake dough
with a moderate level of consistent heat from
both below and above.

c.   The fry pan can be placed directly on a bed of
coals or on a very low flame from a stove. Heat
from above is supplied by placing hot coals
(and/or a twiggy fire) on the fry-pan lid.

d.   The fry pan must be placed on a completely
level and stable platform of coals. Caution must
be exercised in setting the pan on two or more
sticks above the coals since the sticks may burn
through and tip the pan into the fire.

e.   Exercise caution with plastic-handled fry pans
by keeping the handle away from excessive heat.

3.   **Stove-top oven/ring pan**
Available commercially for other purposes, a bundt
pan can serve as an oven for use on most common
backpacking stoves.

a.   The oven consists of an aluminum ring pan and
handle assembly which, when placed directly
over the flame of the stove, allows heat to rise
up through the hole in the ring pan.

b.   When the high, spacious lid of the oven is placed
over the ring pan, the stove heat is forced down
and around the dough, baking it from all sides.

c.   Since the stove is already elevated, the oven can be very easily tipped over if not placed on a perfectly level and stable platform which won't be disturbed.

    d.   Since some backpacking stoves do not have pot-holding arms or rods wide enough to completely support the ring pan, it may be necessary to cut an 8-9" ring of tin flashing to place on the stove and underneath the ring pan for stability.

    e.   Be sure the flashing has a hole in the middle large enough to allow the stove's heat to rise unimpeded.

    f.   Stoves used with this type of oven must be able to burn at a very low flame to allow even simmering.

C. **Preparation of Baked Goods**

Basic "bannock" recipe: The following recipe may be used to make a plain, white biscuit-type roll or bread. Virtually all other doughs and breads that are baked with baking powder (versus yeast) use this recipe or one very similar as a foundation. All measurements are approximate.

The ingredients:
3 to 4 cups white flour
½ to 1 cup powdered milk
½ to 1 tbsp. baking powder
pinch of salt
1 cup cold water

    1.   In a large fry pan or billy can, combine ¾ of the total amount of flour with all the salt, powdered milk, and baking powder. Mix these dry ingredients thoroughly.

    2.   The remaining ¼ of the flour will be used for dusting hands and the pan, and for adding to the dough later.

    3.   Add small amounts of water to the dry mix and stir with a serving spoon. Continue adding water and stirring until the dough thickens to a point where stirring is difficult.

    4.   Thoroughly dust hands with flour and sprinkle about a handful of flour on the dough. Using fingers, fists, and knuckles, knead the dough so that all flour mixes thoroughly into the dough.

5. Continue adding flour and kneading until the dough can be picked up and manipulated by hand without sticking to fingers. The dough should be full of lumps but relatively smooth to the touch.

6. Form the dough into the desired shape for baking or frying (balls, loaf, flat breads, etc.). All dough should be completely prepared before starting the baking or frying process.

D. **Baking**

1. **General suggestions for baking on a fire**

   a. For a baking fire, select hardwoods which will produce hot, long lasting coals.

      (1) Maple, oak, and apple are all good baking firewoods.

      (2) Be sure there is a sufficient wood supply.

   b. To bake in the firepit, enlarge one corner of the pit so that it will easily accommodate the fry pan and handle.

      (1) Provide sufficient space for raking coals into the oven area.

      (2) Some cooks make the baking corner of the firepit a very shallow area to avoid reaching down into a hot, deep firepit to check progress.

   c. Baking over a fire is usually most efficient if performed by two people. One person can start and maintain the fire, while a second person can prepare the baked goods.

   d. Baking platform. Many cooks prefer not to bake directly in the same firepit where other cooking is done.

      (1) To prepare a baking platform, make a low mound of mineral soil adjacent to the firepit which will serve as a baking area.

      (2) Generally, it is best if the platform is made up of mineral soil taken from the pit. The platform should be built so that it affords easy access to hot coals from the fire and stability for the fry-pan oven.

      (3) By hollowing out a small depression in the top of the earthen platform, coals can be placed in the depression, and the oven then placed directly upon them. Some

cooks, fearing that direct contact with coals may burn the dough, place relatively "green" sticks on either side of the depression so that the oven rests upon them, setting the oven about ½ inch above the coals.

e. A small shovel (and a pair of gloves) is necessary for moving coals to and from the oven area.

f. Whether baking in the firepit or on a platform, the temperature of baking coals should be regulated to maintain an even temperature.

    (1) The temperature for baking can best be determined by holding an open hand about 6 inches above the coals. It should feel hot, but not searing.

    (2) Coals beneath the oven should be changed once or twice every ½ hour during the baking time.

    (3) Coals on top of the oven should be maintained at a higher temperature and therefore changed more frequently.

    (4) Coals should be distributed as uniformly as possible around the bottom of the oven so that baking is done evenly. If this is not possible, rotating the oven every few minutes may be necessary.

g. At no time should baked goods be exposed to open flames, as this will virtually guarantee burned goods.

h. Minimize "peeking" inside the oven since cold air can increase the possibility of "fallen" dough.

2. **Baking on the stove**

Baking on the stove is generally easier and quicker than using a campfire, although many experienced outdoor cooks find it less aesthetically satisfying.

a. **Using the fry-pan oven**

    (1) Dough can be baked using the fry-pan oven on the stove over a very low flame.

    (2) A small hot "twiggy" fire can be built on top of the oven lid to provide heat from above.

    (3) To avoid burning the bottom of baked goods, the fry pan should be well greased (with oil or margarine) and dusted with flour before baking.

(4) The stove should be brought to a consistently low flame that can be maintained throughout the baking time.
 b. **Using the ring bundt pan**
(1) As with the fry-pan oven, the ring bundt pan must be thoroughly greased before used for baking.
(2) Make sure the stove and ring bundt pan assembly is completely level so that ingredients do not bubble over the edge or into the middle hole and extinguish the fire.
3. **Making "fry" breads**
 a. Fry-pan breads are another type of baked good popular on the trail. Fry breads are prepared with the same basic "bannock" recipe.
 b. Once the dough is prepared, small handfuls are flattened into round or oblong shapes similar in size and shape to a pancake.
 c. If desired, these "palm breads" can then be filled with a tasty morsel (e.g., cheese, pepperoni, fruit, vegetables), then rolled into a ball and fried. Otherwise, they can be fried flat and used in lieu of sliced bread.
 d. Margarine or vegetable oil both work well for frying. Make sure that oil is hot enough before starting to fry (a drop of water will sizzle when dropped into the correct temperature oil).
 e. Generally, smaller fry breads cook more thoroughly than larger, thicker ones.
 f. Fry breads should be evenly browned on all sides, cooled, then served. Plain fry breads rolled in white or brown sugar make excellent doughnuts.

IV. **INSTRUCTIONAL STRATEGIES & MATERIALS**
 A. **Timing**
1. This class is usually conducted during the latter part of the first week or early part of the second week of instruction.
2. Classes in "Food Identification," "Stove Operation," "Fire Building," "Fire Site Preparation and Care," and "Introductory Cooking" are obvious prerequisites.

B. **Strategies**
1. This class is most commonly taught as a lecture/ demonstration. Instructors can actually go through the entire procedure of dough preparation and baking of both fry bread and traditionally baked goods.
2. To avoid confusion among students, it is usually advisable to limit the presentation to demonstrating one fry bread sample and one oven baked sample.
3. An efficient time-line for this particular lesson might be:
   a. Introduce all baking tools and utensils.
   b. Demonstrate mixing the basic dough.
   c. Start oven-baked product on fire or stove.
   d. Demonstrate and cook fry breads while oven-baked product is baking.
   e. Conclude with a taste test and discussion of recipe alternatives.
4. This class is frequently taught right before lunch or dinner so that the students may put their newly discovered knowledge to immediate use.
5. For additional recipes and ideas, see *NOLS Cookery* or similar publication.

C. **Materials**
1. Fry pan and lid
2. Stove-top oven
3. Stove
4. Existing fire
5. Bowl
6. Water
7. Billy can
8. Spoon
9. Spatula
10. Ingredients (depending on recipes):
    Salt
    Flour
    Milk
    Baking powder
    Sugar
    Misc. spices
    Cheese, pepperoni, dried fruit, etc.

30. Granola Preparation

I. **GOAL**: To have participants demonstrate an ability to prepare granola as a breakfast or trail snack.

II. **OBJECTIVES**:
   A. Participants will properly identify and use the cooking equipment and utensils necessary to prepare granola.
   B. Participants will be able to identify and list the correct ingredients for the preparation of granola.
   C. Participants will demonstrate an ability to prepare a batch of granola suitable for consumption.

III. **CONTENT**:
   A. **Cooking Tools and Utensils**
      Participants should be introduced to each of the following issued cooking tools and utensils:
      1. **Fry pan with lid**
         a. Usually 8-10 inches in diameter. Teflon coating helps eliminate the problem of food sticking to the pan while frying and greatly aids in clean-up.
         b. Pot grips should be used for holding pans over the stove or fire.
      2. **Tote oven**: May be used to fry or bake on either a fire or stove.
      3. **Hard plastic serving spoon**
      4. **Plastic or metal spatula**
      5. **Collapsible plastic water jug or nylon water sack**
      6. **Metal or Lexan plastic cup, bowl, and spoon**: Issued as personal eating gear. May also be used for mixing sauces, pastes, etc.
      7. **Cotton gloves**: Issued to protect hands from excessive drying and cracking when working with fire. They also serve well as pot holders.
      8. **Storage bags**: Cotton/polyester bags used for storing pots, pans, billy can, or utensils. Particularly

© 1992
The Wilderness Education Association
P.O. Box 89
Saranac Lake, New York 12983
(518) 891-2915 ext. 254

helpful in keeping pack contents clean once pots and pans become covered in soot.

B. **Granola Preparation**
1. **Assemble all ingredients** and utensils required for granola preparation prior to lighting the stove.
    a. **Tools and utensils**
        (1) Stove, fuel, matches
        (2) Fry pan and lid
        (3) Spatula
        (4) Pot grips
        (5) Cotton gloves
        (6) Cup, bowl, spoon
        (7) Billy can
    b. **Ingredients**
        (1) Rolled oats (oatmeal)
        (2) Fruits of choice: raisins, dates, apricots, coconut, etc., chopped into bite-size pieces.
        (3) Nuts of choice: almonds, peanuts, sunflower seeds, cashews, etc.
        (4) Sweeteners of choice: honey, brown sugar, white sugar.
        (5) Margarine
        (6) Salt
        (7) Peanut butter (optional)
        (8) M & M's (optional)
        (9) Powdered milk: mixed with water to serve with cold cereal.
2. **Start stove** (see "Stove Operation" lesson plan).
3. **Sterilize utensils** (see "Introductory Cooking" lesson).
4. **Cooking procedure**
    a. Melt 3-4 tablespoons of margarine in a fry pan.
    b. Add oatmeal, stir, and brown.
    c. Add a pinch of salt.
    d. Add nuts and brown.
    e. Add sweeteners to taste. Allow sugars to melt and mix with other ingredients.
    f. Add fruits.
    g. Continue to fry until mixture is browned and toasted to preference.
5. Can serve warm or cool with milk as a cereal, or allow to cool, then bag and use as a trail snack.

IV. INSTRUCTIONAL STRATEGIES & MATERIALS:

A. Timing
This class is usually taught on the first morning as a preparatory lesson for the first breakfast.

B. Strategies
1. This class is often taught in conjunction with the "Stove Operation" class.
2. This is effectively taught in a lecture/demonstration format. The instructor can perform the whole procedure and then participants can immediately go and prepare their own granola for breakfast. Instructors should visit each kitchen/cooking area to assist.
3. If a large enough central area is available, this class could be taught in a step-by-step approach and participants can actually prepare their meal with the instructor as the lesson is taught. One instructor can teach while another circulates among cook groups offering assistance.

C. Materials
1. Fry pan and/or tote oven
2. Pot grips
3. Serving spoon
4. Spatula
5. Water jug or sack
6. Cup, bowl, and spoon
7. Water bottle
8. Cotton gloves
9. Storage sacks
10. Stove, fuel, matches
11. Ingredients:
    a. Oats
    b. Dried fruits of choice (raisins, dates, apricots, coconut, etc.)
    c. Nuts of choice (almonds, peanuts, sunflower seeds, cashews, etc.)
    d. Sweeteners of choice (honey, white sugar, brown sugar)
    e. Margarine
    f. Salt
    g. Peanut butter
    h. Powdered milk

31. Introductory Cooking

I. **GOAL**: To have participants gain the background knowledge necessary to cook meals for themselves and their tent partners.

II. **OBJECTIVES**:
   A. Participants will demonstrate an ability to establish a safe and well-organized kitchen/cooking area.
   B. Participants will know how to use the basic cooking utensils correctly.
   C. Participants will be able to list some fundamental guidelines for success as a novice cook.
   D. Participants will explain the importance of sterilizing utensils before eating.

III. **CONTENT**:
   A. **Safety in the Kitchen/Cooking Area**
      1. The kitchen/cooking area should be located well away from tents, packs, sleeping bags, or other combustible nylon items to prevent sparks from the cooking fire from igniting or damaging equipment.
      2. Whether a stove or cooking fire is used, a 3-5 foot circular "safe" area should be created around it.
         a. No one should walk through, reach over, or horseplay near the fire or stove in the "safe" area.
         b. Only those directly involved in food preparation should work in the "safe" area.
         c. The cooking area should be located in an area free from natural hazards that may trip, poke, or otherwise hinder the cook from working safely around the cooking area.
         d. The cook should designate a comfortable spot to sit near the fire or stove so that he or she may work without constantly shifting around the flames.

© 1992
The Wilderness Education Association
P.O. Box 89
Saranac Lake, New York 12983
(518) 891-2915 ext. 254

e. After the stove has been filled, fuel bottles should be closed securely and removed from the cooking area.

3. Sterilize eating utensils before eating.

a. Sterilizing eating utensils minimizes the chance of intestinal illness due to bacterial growth which may occur between use. Sterilizing is senseless *after* meals because utensils become contaminated when packed.

b. To conserve fuel when cooking on stoves, designate one or two cook groups as "sterilization stations."

c. If cooking on fires, each firepit can have a sterilization pot.

4. Use gloves and/or pot grips when handling hot items.

5. Hot liquids and hot grease must be given special consideration as potential safety hazards.

a. When pouring from a billy can or fry pan, the pouring motion should be directed at a 180° angle away from the pourer.

b. Hot liquids should not be poured into a hand-held container. Instead, containers should be placed on a flat, stable platform, or on the ground.

6. Remove pots that contain boiling food from the stove *before stirring* to prevent accidentally dumping dinner or scalding the cook.

7. Remove pots from the fire before adding food. This prevents plastic bags from burning and minimizes the chance of scalding arms and hands.

8. Do not pass hot items over another person. It may result in severe burns, especially to the ankles and feet.

9. When cooking over a fire, a water-filled billy can should be kept handy for dousing flames or watering the fringes of the firesite.

10. When using a pack stove, an empty billy can should be handy for inverting over the stove to smother a "flare-up."

11. Cooks must be particularly aware of potential dangers such as loose clothing or long hair which may burn around fires or stoves.

a. Long sleeves should be rolled up.

b. Nylon windpants or wind breakers should be removed or protected from heat and sparks.

c.   Long hair should be tied back and kept out of the face and away from flames.

12. Use a hard surface to cut bread, cheese, pepperoni, or other items, rather than using a leg or hands.

13. When using a knife, cut away from oneself.

B. **Cooking Tools and Utensils**

Participants should be introduced to each of the following issued cooking tools and utensils:

1.   **#10 "Billy can"**: a large tin can used for all boiling. Also serves for carrying water, washing clothes and body, or smothering flames on a "flared-up" stove.

2.   **Pot grips**

3.   **Fry pan/tote oven**

4.   **Stove-top oven/ring pan and stabilizing tin**

    a.   The stove-top oven is used for baking on top of the pack stove.

    b.   The stabilizing tin is a circular piece of aluminum flashing material with a hole in the middle. This 8" diameter tin is placed on top of the stove to help stabilize the ring pan oven while baking.

5.   **Hard plastic serving spoon**

6.   **Plastic or metal spatula**

7.   **Collapsible plastic water jug or nylon water sack**

    a.   For carrying and storing water at the campsite.

    b.   Usually holds two to three gallons of water.

8.   **Metal or hard plastic Lexan cup, bowl, and spoon**

    a.   Issued as personal eating gear and may also be used for mixing sauces, pastes, etc.

    b.   Should be submersed in boiling water for sterilization.

9.   **Wide-mouth plastic quart bottle**

    a.   Should be leak proof and able to withstand immersion in boiling water for sterilization.

    b.   Holds water for the trail; may also be used in food preparation.

10. **Cotton gloves**

Issued to protect hands from excessive drying and cracking when working with fire. They also serve as pot holders.

11. **Storage bags**
    Cotton/polyester bags can be used for storing
    stoves, pots, pans, billy cans, or utensils. They are
    particularly helpful in keeping pack contents clean
    once pots and pans become covered in soot.

C. **Organization of the Kitchen Area**
   1. The kitchen area is an area for preparing food. It
      should be separate and distinct from the cooking
      area in order to minimize the danger around the
      stove or fire.
   2. All utensils, pots, and pans required for cooking a
      meal should be organized and laid out in an orderly
      fashion in the cooking area.
      a. Ensolite pads, jackets, or stuff sacks laid on the
         ground can function as "tablecloths" and help
         keep utensils clean and organized.
      b. Cooks should be encouraged to put all utensils
         back in place after each use. This helps avoid
         confusion while cooking and prevents the loss
         of equipment. Pot grips and spoons in
         particular, have a tendency to get lost.
   3. All ingredients required for preparing a meal should
      be organized in the "kitchen" area located at least a
      few feet away from the cooking area.
      a. Ingredients used in meal preparation should be
         removed from the food bag and arranged on a
         "tablecloth."
      b. All food bags that will be used for preparing a
         meal should be opened beforehand to allow
         easy access.
      c. Some cooks like to arrange ingredients in the
         order that they will be needed and replace each
         item in the food bag after use. This maintains
         organization and helps prevent doubling
         ingredients in the pot.
   4. All special preparations for the meal should be
      complete before lighting the stove. This will
      conserve fuel and prevent the need for hasty
      scrambling at the last minute around a lighted stove.

D. **Guidelines For Novice Cooks**
The following is a list of problems typically encountered by novice cooks and suggestions on avoiding them (Simer & Sullivan, 1983):

1. **Burnt food**
    a. Cook on low heat.
    b. Stir constantly.
    c. Be sure there is sufficient water and add more as necessary.
    d. Keep pots clean to minimize the chance of food sticking to the bottom.

2. **Bland vs. overspiced food**
    a. Use salt to bring out the flavor of foods but be careful not to use too much; meals with too much salt are inedible. Add a pinch at a time and taste before adding more.
    b. Experiment with spices one at a time. If four spices are mixed in and the meal tastes terrible, it is hard to tell which spice was the culprit.
    c. Pour the spice into a spoon or hand and then into the pot. Don't pour it directly into the pot or more spice may end up in the meal than planned.
    d. Taste food before spicing – it may not need any.
    e. As part of good expedition behavior, it is important to respect tentpartner's wishes if he or she does not like a certain spice. Spices can always be added to individual portions before eating.

3. **Overdone food**
    Time the meal properly. Add the dehydrated items first and let them rehydrate for 10-15 minutes. Add pastas next and thickeners last.

4. **Lumpy food**
    Thoroughly mix powders (in a cup or bowl) before adding to the pot. Add a little water at a time – it is easy to add more water, but hard to take it away.

5. **High elevations**
    Due to lower atmospheric pressure, cooking times will vary. Water boils away at a lower temperature without reaching 212°F (100°C) so foods don't get as hot.

E. **Dishwashing**
1. Utensils and cookware should be cleaned well away from water sources.
2. Properly dispose of food wastes. (See "Food Waste Disposal" lesson.)
3. If abrasives are necessary, use dead pine needles, spruce twigs, or other natural litter as scouring pads, which should be burned or packed out after use.
4. Pots with stuck or burnt food on the inside can be soaked overnight. By morning the inside will have softened up and will be easier to clean. In bear country, pots should be cleaned immediately after use.
5. Rinse water must be carefully disposed of using appropriate practices for the area. (See "Food Waste Disposal" lesson.)
6. The use of soap is discouraged because it is not necessary and can lead to intestinal illness. Dishwashing soaps are designed for hot water and do not rinse well in cold water.

IV. **INSTRUCTIONAL STRATEGIES & MATERIALS:**
A. **Timing**
1. This course is best taught within the first few days or in a pre-course shakedown to give participants the ability to identify their food and cook.
2. Participants should be encouraged to experiment and be creative in their cooking.

B. **Strategies**
1. This class is often taught in a lecture/discussion format, although it can also be taught in conjunction with "Food Identification" or "Frying and Baking."
2. In grizzly bear country or country where brown bears present a problem:
   a. Prepare and cook food close to a fire ring.
   b. Never eat or store food in a tent. The odor will remain even after the food is gone.
   c. Don't sleep in clothing that has been soiled with food, stored with food, or worn while cooking. Store containers that have or have had food, drink mix, or fuel, away from the tent at night.

C. **Materials**
1. A good kitchen/cooking area
2. Billy can
3. Fry pan/tote oven
4. Stove-top oven and stabilizing tin
5. Serving spoon
6. Spatula
7. Water jug or sack
8. Cup, bowl, and spoon
9. Water bottle
10. Cotton gloves
11. Storage bags for utensils and pots
12. Food bags
13. Stove and/or fire

32. Yeast Baking

I. **GOAL**: To have participants demonstrate an ability to produce well-made baked goods using yeast dough.

II. **OBJECTIVES**:
   A. Participants will be able to describe some of the advantages of baking with yeast on the trail.
   B. Participants will be able to explain in simple terms how yeast works as a baking ingredient.
   C. Participants will be able to correctly identify and use the equipment and cooking ingredients associated with yeast baking.
   D. Participants will be able to describe some basic recipes that may be used to make yeast-baked goods.
   E. Participants will be able to describe and correctly demonstrate all the steps and procedures for making yeast bread.

III. **CONTENT**:
   A. **The Joys of Yeast Baking**
      1. **Good food**
         Baking with yeast adds an almost infinite variety of baked goods to the backcountry larder. Good yeast breads, buns, doughnuts, etc. are always a welcome addition to the menu.
      2. **Good morale**
         Baking with yeast can be an extremely relaxing, self-satisfying, and productive activity for the individual or the entire group. The slow, patient pace associated with rising dough and baking bread allows for moments of contemplative solitude or quiet group conversation unhurried by the demands of the daily itinerary.

© 1992
The Wilderness Education Association
P.O. Box 89
Saranac Lake, New York 12983
(518) 891-2915 ext. 254

3. **Good companionship**
   Baking with or for other members of the expedition is a superb way to develop or bind friendships.

B. **The Science of Yeast Baking**
   1. Yeast are one-celled organisms that come alive and metabolize if given the proper environment — warm water and a food source of sugar or starch.
      a. Water temperature must not be too hot or too cool. Optimum temperature for yeast growth is 110°F (43°C) or water slightly hot to the touch.
      b. Yeast can feed on white or brown sugar directly, or make sugar from other starches. In either case, when the proper host environment is provided, the yeast begins to metabolize and release CO_2 gas which, when trapped by the gluten fibers in the dough, causes the dough to rise.
   2. In order to make bread that rises well, flour with high concentrations of gluten should be used. When the moist dough is kneaded, the gluten fibers in the dough become very elastic and almost rubbery. These elastic fibers help to form a surface which traps the CO_2 gas emitted by the yeast.
      a. Whole wheat flour is high in gluten content and should be included in most bread recipes for beginners.
      b. Combining whole wheat and white flour makes a good beginner's dough.

C. **Preparation for Yeast Baking**
   1. **The tools**
      a. Backpacking stove, fuel, and matches. Yeast baking on a good backpacking stove is a joy, since temperature levels can be maintained at a constant level over long periods.
      b. Billy can
      c. Large spoon, cup, or bowl
      d. Sleeping pad (except in bear country). Preferably a clean, closed-cell pad.
      e. Stove-top oven or ring pan with lid

2. **The ingredients** (See *NOLS Cookery* for additional recipes.)

    a.   **The basic NOLS yeast dough recipe:**

        3 to 4 cups flour
        2 tsp. salt
        2 tbsp. sugar
        1¾ cups water in a billy can (approx. 1 inch)
        1 tbsp. quick-rise yeast

    b.   **North Country Community College recipe:**
        makes 2 loaves of sweet, whole wheat bread.

        1 tbsp. quick-rise yeast
        1 tsp. sugar
        ½ cup warm water (110°F/43°C)
        ½ cup powdered milk solution (powdered milk and water)
        1½ tbsp. margarine
        2 tbsp. cooking oil
        ½ tbsp. salt
        ¾ cup honey
        ½ cup hot water
        2 cups whole wheat flour
        2 to 3 cups white flour

D. **The Baking Process**

1. Organize the kitchen area and ingredients as for any major cooking adventure. Be sure all ingredients are readily accessible.

2. Heat 2 cups of water on the stove. Pour ½ cup of this hot water into a cup or bowl. Swish the water around until it cools to approximately 110°F/43°C (just hot to the touch). Add yeast and 1 tsp. of sugar to the water and stir gently. Allow this yeast solution to stand about 5 minutes. The solution should show gas bubble formations within a few minutes and develop a froth if the yeast is fresh and properly metabolizing.

3. If there are no signs of gas activity, check the water temperature. If the water is too cool, the yeast has not yet been activated — add warm water. If the water is too hot, the yeast has probably been killed — start over.

4. While the yeast is metabolizing, prepare the liquid ingredients. In a billy can, mix the milk solution, honey, salt, margarine, and hot water. Stir the mix until the margarine is thoroughly melted.

5. When the yeast solution is ready (frothy) and the contents of the billy can have cooled below 110°F/ 43°C, pour the yeast solution into the billy can.

6. Add whole wheat flour and 1½ cups of white flour to the mix. Do not pour all of the flour called for by the recipe into the mix at once. At least ¾ of the white flour should be set aside for powdering hands, dusting the kneading surface, and for adding to the mix.

7. Once the wet and dry ingredients are mixed, stir vigorously with a large spoon until the mix becomes too thick to stir. Add small sprinkles of flour to the dough until it becomes thick enough and dry enough to be picked up by hand.

8. Dust hands with white flour. Also dust a section of a closed-cell sleeping pad or a large flat rock which will be used for kneading the dough.

9. Pick up the dough and place on the floured hard surface. Knead the dough (pushing, spreading, and folding dough over with heel of hands) for 8-10 minutes to form air pockets and mix ingredients. Add additional flour to hands and knead surface to keep the dough from sticking.

10. Continue to knead the dough until it becomes springy and resists further manipulation. The surface of well-kneaded dough will become smooth and silky, "like a baby's bottom."

11. Shape the dough into 1 or 2 loaves and place in a very well-oiled or greased stove-top oven or frying pan. Grease all sides of the loaf, including the top, with oil. Cover the loaf and pan with a moist bandana and place it in the hot sun or near warm coals to rise for 45-60 minutes. (Weather conditions and temperature will greatly affect rising time. Warm, sunny, high pressure days make for excellent baking.)

12. If the loaf is going to be baked in a relatively shallow stove-top oven, the dough should not be allowed to rise above the lip of the bottom pan. Although baking temperatures do kill yeast activity, the dough

will continue to rise dramatically during the early stages of baking. This additional spurt must be accommodated by the oven, or the dough will spill over the pan and burn.

13. Once the dough has risen to the appropriate size, cover with the stove lid and bake for 35-60 minutes over the stove or on an appropriate fire. The bread is done when the surface is golden brown, crisp, and sounds hollow when thumped with a finger.

14. When the bread is done, allow it to cool in the pan for 10-15 minutes. Remove from the oven and allow to cool on a clean surface.

IV. INSTRUCTIONAL STRATEGIES & MATERIALS

A. Timing

1. Yeast baking as a formal class is typically taught around the mid-point of the expedition after participants have thoroughly familiarized themselves with basic techniques of cooking and baking.

2. Ideally, a baking class should be conducted on a layover or rest day so that participants may enjoy the aesthetic rewards of the class as well as good food.

B. Strategies

1. Although yeast baking can be taught one-on-one at any time during the course, the most rewarding type of class for this activity is large group instruction.

2. Assuming there is an area of sufficient size to accommodate the group, participants can be paired up and encouraged to work together during the class. Students can follow the example of an instructor by moving step-by-step through the mixing and baking process.

3. If an area of sufficient size is not available for a large group activity, the class can be taught in a more traditional setting with lecture/demonstration and note-taking. Participants should be encouraged to put their newly acquired knowledge into practice as soon as possible. Naturally, instructors should be available to lend advice and support at each of the cooking sites where yeast baking is being attempted for the first time.

C. **Materials**
1. Backpacking stove, fuel, and matches
2. Billy can
3. Large spoon, cup, or bowl
4. Sleeping pad. Preferably a clean, closed-cell pad
5. Stove-top oven or ring pan with lid
6. Ingredients, depending on recipe:
   - flour (white and/or whole wheat)
   - sweetener (white or brown sugar, and/or honey)
   - water
   - yeast
   - powdered milk
   - margarine
   - cooking oil
   - salt

33. Map Folding

I. **GOAL**: To have participants be able to fold a map for efficient use and storage.

II. **OBJECTIVES**:
   A. Participants will be able to fold a map.
   B. Participants will be able to explain why the map is folded a certain way.
   C. Participants will be able to store a map for protection.

III. **CONTENT**:
   A. **Demonstration of Map Folding**
       1. Fold the map in half lengthwise so that the printed side of the map faces in. (See Figure 33-1.)
       2. Fold back half of one length so that the side map margin aligns with the first fold. (See Figure 33-2.) The printed side should face up and the quadrangle name should show at the bottom. Turn the map over and do the same with the other side of the map.
       3. The map should now be folded in quarters, lengthwise. (The printed side should face out.) Fold the map in half so that the quadrangle names face each other and the top and bottom map margins meet. (See Figure 33-3.)
       4. Fold back one half of each folded half of the map so that the quadrangle names are facing out. (See Figure 33-4.) Turn the map over and do the same on the other side. The quadrangle name should now face out.

© 1992
The Wilderness Education Association
P.O. Box 89
Saranac Lake, New York 12983
(518) 891-2915 ext. 254

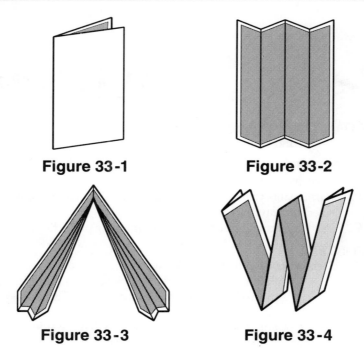

Figure 33-1　　　　　　**Figure 33-2**

Figure 33-3　　　　　　**Figure 33-4**

B. **Why the Map is Folded This Way**
1. It allows easy identification of the map.
2. The original creases can be used to refold the map. Also, any quad (section) of the map can be seen at one time.
3. Most maps that are folded this way will fit into a shirt pocket.

C. **Map Storage**
1. A plastic bag with an overhand knot or a zippered plastic bag provide effective and inexpensive methods of storing maps. Reinforce the need to keep the map in the bag nearly all the time, even when it is not raining. Perspiration as well as any other type of moisture will rapidly shorten the life of the map.
2. A more effective way to protect a map from moisture is to seal it with a commercial waterproofing agent such as Aquaseal or Thompson's Water Seal.

228

IV. INSTRUCTIONAL STRATEGIES & MATERIALS:

A. **Timing**

This is an excellent lesson for a teachable moment. It is also appropriate for student instruction, as it is a relatively simple lesson but requires good communication skills and the ability to give a demonstration.

B. **Strategies**
1. Walk through each step with the participants (i.e., make one fold, then have them make the fold). Make sure they are following each step — don't get ahead.
2. Have participants put their names on their maps so they don't get them mixed up with others'.
3. Ask participants why they think the map is folded this way.

C. **Materials**
1. Maps
2. Plastic bags and/or map seal

229

34. Map Interpretation

I.   **GOAL**: To have participants interpret a map effectively for safe travel in the backcountry.

II. **OBJECTIVES**:
   A.   Participants will be able to define and describe the function of a topographic map.
   B.   Participants will be able to identify and properly locate nine features of a topographic map.
   C.   Participants will be able to identify and properly describe the function of five elevation designations.

III. **CONTENT**:
   A.   **General Background**
      1.   A map is "a reduced representation of a portion of the surface of the earth" (Kjellstrom, 1976, p. 8).
      2.   A topographic map is a map that shows the three dimensional features of the land's surface in two dimensions. "Topos" = place; "Graphein" = to write or draw (Kjellstrom, 1976).
      3.   Where to purchase maps
         a.   U.S. Geological Survey, Denver, Colorado
         b.   Local sporting goods stores

   B.   **Map Margin Information**
      Identify each of the following:
      1.   Name of the map
      2.   Names of adjacent maps
      3.   Location of the map on the earth's surface
         a.   Longitude, note meridians
         b.   Latitude, note parallels
      4.   Date of the map – note possible changes that may have occurred since the map was drawn and field tested.
      5.   Map scale/series – note how the scale is drawn.

© 1992
The Wilderness Education Association
P.O. Box 89
Saranac Lake, New York 12983
(518) 891-2915 ext. 254

a. **Scale ratio**
inches/cm. on map = inches/cm. in the field
(1) **1:24,000**
This map is good for detailed study of a small area.
1 inch = 2,000 feet in field.
Approximately 2½ inches = 1 mile.
1 cm. = 240 m., 4 cm. = 1 km.
(2) **1:25,000**
Used in metric series, similar to 1:24,000 scale.
1 cm. = 250 m
(3) **1:62,500**
Good general purpose map.
Approximately 1 inch = 1 mile in field.
1 cm. = 625 m., 1.5 cm. = 1 km.

b. **Series**
(1) **15" (minute) series**
This map covers a section of the earth's surface 15" of longitude x 15" of latitude. Note longitude and latitude marks on map to confirm size.
(2) **7½" series**
Note that it takes four 7½" maps to equal a 15" map.
(3) **7½" x 15" series**
Metric series found only in a few areas of the United States.

C. **General Map Details**
Identify the location of each detail on a sample map.
1. **Map symbols**
a. **Cultural symbols** – symbols of human-made objects. These are represented by the color **black**.
(1) Roads
(2) Railroads
(3) Churches
(4) Trails
(5) Buildings
(6) Cemeteries
(7) Bridges
(8) Schools
(9) Quarries/mines

b. **Water symbols** – represented by the color **blue.**
       (1) Lakes
       (2) Streams
          (a) On 7½" maps, for a stream width of more than 40 ft. (12 m.), both shores are shown.
          (b) On 15" maps, for a stream width of more than 80 ft. (24 m.), both shores are shown.
       (3) Springs
       (4) Marshes/swamps
    c. **Map directions**
       (1) True north
          This is the north that is shown on a map.
       (2) Magnetic north
          This is the north that attracts the compass needle. Subsequent navigation lessons ("Compass: An Introduction" and "Combining the Map and Compass") will discuss the two norths and declination in more detail.
       (3) Place name designations
          Note the different styles of lettering used for area names, elevation figures, political boundaries, etc.
  2. **Elevation markings** – these are represented by the color **brown**.
    a. **Contour lines**
      "An imaginary line on the ground along which every point is at the same height above sea level" (Kjellstrom, 1976, p. 23). Note the altitude numbers located along some contour lines.
       (1) **Index contour**
          Heavier brown contour lines usually spaced at 100 ft. elevation intervals.
       (2) **Intermediate contours**
          The contour lines between index contours.
       (3) **Contour interval**
          "The distance in height between one contour line and the one next to it" (Kjellstrom, 1976, p. 23). Intervals vary from map to map.

b. **Contour shapes**
   (1) Hills & mountains
   (2) Passes
   (3) Steep areas
   (4) Flat areas
c. **Depression contours**
d. **Interpreting elevation change**
   (1) Contours forming V's generally point uphill.
   (2) Streams which come together forming V's generally point downhill.
e. **Benchmarks**
   "BM" represents the location of a marker in the field where altitude or distance has been verified. The number next to "BM" indicates altitude.
   (1) Horizontal
   (2) Vertical

IV. **INSTRUCTIONAL STRATEGIES & MATERIALS:**
   A. **Timing**
   Map skills may be introduced to participants almost immediately while traveling the first few days of the course. More formalized classes are usually taught in conjunction with a trailless hike or mountain climb when skills can be applied immediately.

   B. **Strategies**
   1. Early map skills can be developed along the trail and during breaks. Calling attention to prominent topographic features and then locating them on the map arouses interest, introduces map terminology, and encourages participants to become more aware of their natural surroundings. Asking participants to predict upcoming terrain features encourages them to continue map use on the trail. Asking participants to measure distance traveled encourages awareness of map scale and builds a base of experience for later time control plan development.
   2. Formalized map classes may be a combination of lecture and discussion depending upon the extent of participant knowledge. The class should focus on a general overview of all map features and their identification on sample maps. Instructors may ask participants to conduct a theoretical journey across the map and describe the identifiable map features,

obstacles, or land forms that they will encounter along the way.

3. More advanced map skills are best developed in practice on a trailless hike where participants must concentrate on observing terrain features in order to follow progress on their maps. Treeless mountain tops make excellent classroom sites for understanding contouring, distance, and how terrain may have changed over time. Ask participants to orient their maps without the use of their compass, thereby using the opportunity to identify prominent land features.

4. Use the knuckles to describe contours. Draw lines on knuckles with the hand in a fist, then open the hand to show how the lines look on a topographic map.

5. Use a sand pile to describe contours.

C. **Materials**
1. A map for at least every two participants. All maps should be of the same area.
2. Blank paper and pen. In lieu of a blackboard, this can come in handy to help describe map symbols and features.

35. Compass: An Introduction

I.   GOAL: To have participants use a compass effectively for safe travel in the backcountry.

II. OBJECTIVES:
  A. Participants will be able to explain the function of a compass in finding direction in the field.
  B. Participants will be able to identify and properly describe the function of all parts of a compass.
  C. Participants will be able to explain and properly demonstrate the technique of taking a field bearing.

III. CONTENT:
  A. **Concept of "Direction"**
    1. Direction is defined as the line of travel or sight from point A (present location) to point B (destination).
    2. Direction is expressed in terms of the 360 degrees of a circle.
      a. Present location is assumed to be the center of the circle.
      b. Any direction can be expressed in terms of the degrees of an angle measured clockwise from a point at the top of the circle to the point on the circumference representing the direction.
      c. For two or more people to describe a direction to each other accurately, they must establish a common "top of the circle" from which degrees will be measured. True North has been universally identified as the top of the circle. *Give examples of directions N, S, E, and W in degrees.*

  B. **Parts of the compass** (based on the Silva™ Polaris Type 7 and similar compasses)
    1. **Base plate**
      a. The rectangular, transparent piece of plastic upon which all compass parts rest.

235

b. This plate typically has millimeter and inch markings along the edge for measuring.

c. The edges of the base plate are parallel to the "direction of travel arrow," which is engraved upon it.

2. **"Direction of travel" arrow**

a. Engraved arrow on the base plate which runs from the edge of the compass housing to one end of the base plate.

b. Compass bearings or degree readings are taken from the point where the base of the direction of travel arrow touches the numbers on the edge of the compass housing.

c. Whether using in the field or on a map, the direction of travel arrow must always point toward the intended destination.

3. **Compass housing**

a. Circular, rotating rim found in the middle of the base plate.

b. It has the initials of the four cardinal points, N, S, E, and W on the upper rim, and degree lines on the outer rim.

c. Most compasses have lines representing increments of 2° of angle with every twentieth degree numbered. Some smaller compasses have only 5° increments.

4. **Magnetic needle**

a. The magnetic needle is suspended on a bearing in the middle of the liquid-filled, plastic-cased housing.

b. This needle points to Magnetic North when the compass is held steady and level.

5. **Orienting arrow and orienting/meridian lines**

a. Usually in blue or white, these are represented by the outline of an arrow. They are also the parallel lines engraved in the plastic bottom of the housing.

b. The arrow points directly to the 360°/0° mark on the compass housing.

c. The compass is said to be "oriented" or "boxed" when the compass housing is turned so that the magnetic needle lies directly over the orienting arrow, and both the arrow and

the needle simultaneously point to the letter
"N" on the compass housing rim.

   d.   The orienting lines run parallel to the orienting
arrow and are used in establishing map bearings.

C. **Function of the Compass**

   1.   The magnetic needle of the compass always points
to Magnetic North. This provides a constant and
common reference point (360°/0°) from which all
directional degree designations may be measured.

   2.   By facing True North, then pointing to an intended
destination (B in Figure 35-1), an imaginary angle is
formed by the line pointing True North and the line
pointing to the destination. The meeting point of
these two legs of the angle is the observer's present
location (A in Figure 35-1).

   3.   The primary function of the compass is to assist the
backcountry traveler in establishing the direction of
North and thereby measuring the angle or "bearing"
of the intended line of travel to the destination.

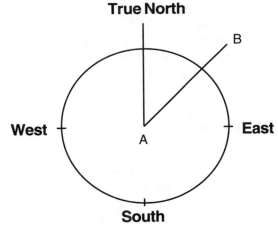

Figure 35-1 The Compass Bearing

D. **Using a "Field Bearing"**

A "field bearing" is the angle of the line of travel established when the compass alone is used to sight a
destination in the field.

   1.   **Taking a field bearing**

      a.   Squarely face the distant point which is the
intended destination.

b.   Hold the compass level in the palm of one hand and at mid-chest height with the direction of travel arrow pointed directly at the destination.

c.   Orient or "box" the compass by turning the compass housing until the magnetic needle rests squarely over the orienting arrow.

(1)   Both the magnetic needle and the orienting arrow should point to "N."

(2)   Make sure to turn only the compass housing — do not move the base plate or turn your body away from the direction of travel to your intended destination.

d.   Once the compass is oriented and the magnetic needle comes to rest, read the degree marking on the rim of the compass housing where it intersects the tail of the direction of travel arrow and where it usually says, "Read Bearing Here." This degree reading is the "field bearing" which should be written down for reference and followed during travel to the destination.

e.   When taking bearings, be sure the compass is not exposed to metal objects, iron deposits, or magnetic fields which may cause the magnetic needle to function improperly.

E.   **Following a Field Bearing**

1.   Once a field bearing is established, travel may proceed along the line of travel on a relatively straight course (depending upon the terrain) by following the direction of travel arrow.

2.   Since the sight of the original destination point may be lost during travel, it is important to start the trek by spotting a clearly visible landmark that is nearby and is on the same bearing as the destination.

a.   By moving from one known landmark, checking the bearing, then moving on to the next sighted landmark, the traveler can proceed along the line of travel without constantly following the exact path indicated by the compass.

b.   This "leap frog" method of travel allows the traveler to circumvent hazards or obstacles while still holding to the correct line of travel.

3.   Once the destination is reached, a return route may be easily established by adding or subtracting 180° to or from the original bearing. This "back-bearing" just reverses the original line of travel and allows the traveler to proceed back along the original route to the starting point.

IV. INSTRUCTIONAL STRATEGIES & MATERIALS:
A.   **Timing**
This lesson is usually taught after participants have gained some experience with maps and their use.

B.   **Strategies**
1.   Introduction to the compass can start while on the trail with simple exercises that establish the location of North, the general direction of travel along the trail, etc. Compass terminology may also be introduced during breaks.
2.   Early formal classes on the compass should combine lectures and demonstrations with an immediate opportunity for practice. Following instruction in the technique of establishing field and map bearings, participants should immediately apply this knowledge in the surrounding environment by taking bearings on easily visible landmarks and matching them on their maps.
3.   Once participants have gained confidence in taking bearings, a short compass course or simple trailless hike will allow participants to practice following a bearing in the field. Special care should be taken to ensure that the compass course area is completely "safe" so that "disoriented" students cannot get lost. Students should be teamed up so that route determination is a group effort. This allows for mutual teaching, reinforcement, and confidence.

C.   **Materials**
1.   One compass per student
2.   Paper and pen: In lieu of a blackboard, this can be very handy to describe parts and functions of the compass.
3.   Cord
     a.   This can be useful in describing the concept of bearings as angles.
     b.   Ideally, a different color cord could represent a different radius of the angle of a bearing.

36. Combining the Map and Compass

I. **GOAL**: To have participants combine knowledge of map and compass effectively for safe travel in the backcountry.

II. **OBJECTIVES**:
   A. Participants will be able to explain and properly demonstrate how to take a map bearing.
   B. Participants will be able to explain and properly demonstrate how to orient a map with a compass.
   C. Participants will be able to explain and apply declination.
   D. Participants will be able to explain and properly demonstrate how to convert map bearings to field bearings and vice versa.

III. **CONTENT**:
   A. **Philosophy**
   Once experience has been gained with maps and compasses separately, the two skills can be combined to maximize their potential. However, it is important to keep in mind that when used together, both should be relied upon and not one without the other.
   1. Use the map to find easier routes that are close enough to the original bearing and the destination. Don't blindly follow a bearing that goes through swamps and up cliffs.
   2. Don't take the easiest route if it contradicts the bearing.
   3. Generally speaking, when in doubt, rely on the bearing. The terrain can be deceiving while a correct bearing is generally not.

B. **Using Map and Compass**
  1. **Taking a map bearing**
     a. The compass may be used as a protractor when attempting to establish a bearing for travel from one known place on a map to another.
     b. Place the compass on the map with one of the long edges of the base plate connecting the starting point of the trip with the destination. Be sure the "direction of travel" arrow is pointing in the direction of the destination.
     c. Twist the compass housing until the orienting arrow and the meridian lines (or "map aid" lines) within the housing are parallel with the nearest north/south longitudinal line (meridian) on the map.
        (1) The only true North/South lines are those printed on the map margins (and the "ticks" that mark the "neat" lines). It is important for participants to understand that the grid lines on a map are not true North/South meridian lines. It is best to use the edge of the map or any line parallel to the edge for taking a map bearing.
        (2) Be sure the orienting arrow is pointing to True North at the top of the map.
     d. Read the map bearing from the rim of the housing where it intersects with the direction of travel arrow. This reading is called a "map bearing," i.e., the angle measured in degrees formed by a line of travel on a map in relationship to True North (top of map).
     e. Some like to draw parallel north/south lines on the map in pencil to insure accuracy when taking bearings although, as will be seen shortly, a better method may be employed.
  2. **Declination: using a map bearing**
     a. This is a good time to introduce declination because, before understanding how a map bearing can be used in the field as a guide for travel, declination must be taken into consideration.
     b. Declination is the difference, expressed in degrees of an angle, between the location of

True North (as found on a map) and that of
Magnetic North (as shown by a compass)
measured from any given location on the globe.

(1) The declination for any given area is
recorded on the bottom of that area's map.

(2) This measurement must be checked and
accounted for before wilderness travel by
map and compass is undertaken.

c. If, as is the case for much of the eastern U.S.,
Magnetic North is located some degrees west of
the North Pole (True North), then:

(1) **Declination + Map Bearing = Field Bearing**
For instance, in New York State where the
average declination is 14°, that 14° must be
added to any map bearing before it can be
used accurately in the field to find the
way. (The reverse would be done west of
0° declination: Declination - Map Bearing
= Field Bearing.)

(2) **Field Bearing - Declination = Map Bearing**
Again, in New York State with an average
declination of 14°, 14° must be subtracted
from any field bearing before that measurement may be accurately used to find a
location on a topographic map. (The
reverse would be done west of 0°
declination: Field Bearing + Declination =
Map Bearing.) See Figure 36-1.

d. Drawing pencil lines parallel to Magnetic
North/South (i.e., parallel to the margins)
across the map will eliminate the need to add
or subtract when taking map bearings.
However, this method is discouraged until
participants have a thorough understanding of
why and when to add or subtract when taking
map bearings and plotting field bearings.

3. **Orienting a map with the compass**

a. When observing terrain features in the field, it
is frequently helpful to line up the map so that
it faces the same way as the observer. This
lining-up of the features of the map with those
in the field is known as orienting the map.

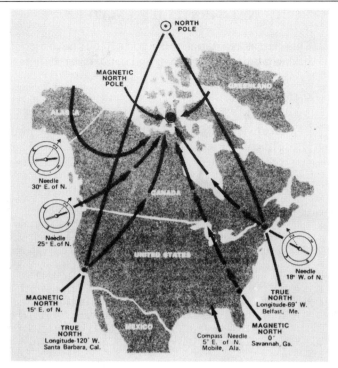

Reprinted by permission from the author
Kjellstrom, "Be Expert with Map and Compass."

Figure 36-1 Declination

b. Orienting the map can be easily accomplished with the compass.

(1) Set the compass "direction of travel" arrow at the appropriate declination for the area.

(2) Place one of the long side edges of the compass base plate along either of the north/south margins of the map. Make sure the "direction of travel" arrow is heading in a northerly direction.

(3) Turn the map, with the compass on it, until the magnetic needle is "boxed" by the orienting arrow. Both the compass and the map are now oriented.

IV. INSTRUCTIONAL STRATEGIES & MATERIALS:

A. **Timing**

This class is best taught after participants have a good understanding of both map and compass and are ready to combine the two.

B. **Strategies**

1. Teaching declination should inspire especially creative efforts from instructors. Since this concept is difficult for some to grasp, instructors should be prepared to use a number of approaches to illustrate the idea.

2. Visual aids (diagrams) and props (colored shoe strings representing True North, Magnetic North, and line of travel) should be employed to help visualize the concept in different ways.

3. Mnemonic phrases help participants remember how to convert map bearings to field bearings (e.g., **FM Stereo = F**ield to **M**ap, **S**ubtract).

4. A skit can be used where participants play the following roles: True North, Magnetic North, the east coast, St. Louis, and California. Angles and declination can be demonstrated by using "St. Louis" as 0°.

C. **Materials**

1. Maps
2. Compasses
3. Visual aids, as needed

37. Route Finding
with Map and Compass

I. **GOAL**: To have participants demonstrate the ability to plan and execute a safe, trailless hike.

II. **OBJECTIVE**:
Participants will be able to discuss and successfully apply compass and map skills to the planning and proper execution of a trailless hike.

III. **CONTENT**:
   A. **Terrain Considerations**
   Once participants have gained some experience and confidence in their map and compass skills, they can plan and attempt a trailless hike.
   1. The safety of the group must be of paramount concern during route planning. Obviously, dangerous obstacles such as cliffs, large rivers, and crevasses should be avoided.
   2. Alternate routes should be planned if these areas or other questionable areas (such as swamps or bogs) are deemed unsafe to travel through.

   B. **Comfort**
   The comfort of the group should be considered in route planning.
   1. How much altitude must be gained?
   2. Is there water available along the route?
   3. How thick might the forests be?
   4. Will the terrain be very wet or insect-ridden?

   C. **Time and Distance**
   It is important to accurately predict how much time will be required to travel the desired distance.

© 1992
The Wilderness Education Association
P.O. Box 89
Saranac Lake, New York 12983
(518) 891-2915 ext. 254

1. **Terrain features**
    Terrain features such as steep terrain, thick woods, and wet swamps all slow down travel time considerably.
2. **Routes**
    Choose routes that ensure that the group has adequate time to accomplish the objective, even if a minor emergency occurs.
3. **Establish guideposts**
    Select routes that allow the traveler to look for clearly identifiable land forms and features to use as guides, minimizing the opportunity for getting lost.
    a. **Handrails**
        (1) Select land features that parallel the line of travel to the left or right.
        (2) If a traveler crosses over a handrail, it should indicate that they have drifted off to the left or right of the chosen path.
    b. **Backstop**
        (1) Select a land form to serve as a "dead end" or "gone too far" barrier.
        (2) Hitting this land form indicates that a turn was missed or the objective was passed.
    c. **Checkpoints**
        (1) Selected land or terrain forms (i.e., checkpoints) along the line of travel can be used to confirm the traveler's exact location.
        (2) These checkpoints can be used frequently to evaluate progress and determine on a map whether or not travel is going as planned. Travelers should use the map to keep constant track of their location.
4. **Altitude gain or loss**
    a. The gain or loss of altitude along a route must be properly estimated in order to make an accurate Time Control Plan and can be another clue about the accuracy of the route chosen.
    b. The group can count contour lines from the starting point to the destination to get an idea of the ruggedness of the terrain (see "Trail Technique: Advanced" for more detail).
5. **Distance**
    a. The distance of the proposed route should be measured using a string and the distance scale.

b. Distance naturally figures into the Time Control Plan.

6. **Time Control Plan**

a. Participants should be encouraged to submit a written estimate of the time it will take to reach the objective.

b. This estimate may be broken down into travel time and rest time if desired.

c. This estimate can help build the participants' base of experiential knowledge.

IV. **INSTRUCTIONAL STRATEGIES & MATERIALS:**

A. **Timing**

1. As their confidence builds, participants should be encouraged to plan and execute progressively more difficult trailless hikes. Planning sessions for trips should include instruction and discussion of the following:

a. Terrain considerations in route planning

b. Identifying potential "handrails," "backstops," and "checkpoints."

c. Altitude loss or gain and counting contour lines

d. Estimating distances

e. Developing Time Control Plans

2. Participants should be encouraged to submit written estimates or predictions for each area of concern. During debriefings, these can be compared to the actual travel experience, which helps build a base of knowledge.

3. Use the concept of an "energy mile" to estimate travel time.

a. The average speed that a group with full packs walks on flat terrain is 2 m.p.h..

b. At altitudes up to 7000 feet, for every 1000 feet of elevation gained, add 1 hour.

c. At altitudes between 7000 feet and 11,000 feet, for every 1000 feet of elevation gained, add $1\frac{1}{2}$ hours.

d. For every 1000 feet of elevation lost, add 30 minutes.

38. Triangulation
with Map and Compass

I. **GOAL**: To have participants triangulate with a map and compass to determine their location.

II. **OBJECTIVE**:
   A. Participants will be able to explain and demonstrate triangulation using a map and compass.

III. **CONTENT**:
   A. **Definition of Triangulation**
      The process of locating an unknown point by using intersecting bearings taken on three known points.

   B. **Steps**
      1. Using a topographic map of the area, positively identify two or three known landmarks that can be seen both in the field and on the map.
      2. Take a field bearing of landmark #1. Write this bearing down and convert it to a map bearing. (Be sure to consider the area's declination.)
      3. Set the compass for the map bearing of landmark #1.
         a. Place the edge of the compass base plate with the "direction of travel" arrow facing landmark #1 on the map.
         b. Keeping the front tip of the base plate on landmark #1, rotate the compass base plate around the landmark until the orienting arrow and the orienting/meridian lines are pointing to True North/South on the map.
         c. Pencil in a line on the map along the compass base plate edge which touches landmark #1. (This line may have to be extended.)
         d. The present location lies somewhere along this bearing.

© 1992
The Wilderness Education Association
P.O. Box 89
Saranac Lake, New York 12983
(518) 891-2915 ext. 254

4. Repeat the same procedure for landmark #2 and landmark #3.
   a. Once all three bearings are recorded on the map, the lines should intersect or at least form a small triangle at some point on the map. This location is the approximate spot from which the three bearings were taken (i.e., the present location).
   b. Participants should not be discouraged if the lines do not meet precisely at some given point. Given the level of sophistication of normal compasses and the participant's skill level, an approximate location should suffice to satisfy the need to know "where we are."

IV. **INSTRUCTIONAL STRATEGIES & MATERIALS:**
   A. **Timing**
      This is an advanced map and compass technique and should be taught once participants have some degree of familiarity with both map and compass.

   B. **Strategies**
      1. Triangulation is best taught on treeless mountain tops or at least in areas of open visibility where clearly distinguishable landmarks can be seen.
      2. For practice, participants can triangulate an already known (present) location.
      3. The instructor can provide bearings to identify a hypothetical "unknown" location on the map.
      4. Participants should attempt to locate their approximate position at some convenient time on a trailless hike using triangulation.

   C. **Materials**
      1. At least one map for every two participants
      2. One compass for each participant
      3. Pencil

39. Emergency Procedures

I. **GOAL**: To have participants understand the considerations in emergency planning, implement specific emergency procedures, and develop a field emergency plan.

II. **OBJECTIVES**:
 A. Participants will be able to list the considerations in the immediate care of the ill or injured beyond administering emergency medical care.
 B. Participants will be able to determine which type of evacuation would be most appropriate in a given situation.
 C. Participants will be able to list post-accident considerations.

III. **CONTENT**:
 A. **Emergency Procedures**
  1. **Definition**: the procedures to be performed at the time of an accident or illness.
  2. **Immediate considerations at the time of the emergency:**
   a. Stop and think. Decisions should not be rushed but carefully thought out within the time limits of the particular emergency.
   b. Delegate authority. The leader should have those who are most qualified take appropriate roles. For example:
    (1) Performance of emergency medical care.
    (2) Secretary – This person should write down times, dates, first aid performed, medicine given the patient, etc.
    (3) Messengers – Those who will run for help if necessary.
    (4) Assistants – Those who may help the rest of the group set up camp or accomplish whatever tasks may need to be completed.

© 1992
The Wilderness Education Association
P.O. Box 89
Saranac Lake, New York 12983
(518) 891-2915 ext. 254

     c. Miscellaneous care of the patient and the group.
        (1) Creating a calm atmosphere
        (2) Tender, loving care for the patient
     d. Does the patient need to be evacuated?
     e. Is outside assistance required?

3. **Considerations in requesting outside assistance**
   a. At least three (preferably four) capable "messengers" should be selected to go request assistance. (Four people is ideal so that if one of the messengers is injured on the way out, one can remain with the injured person and there are still two to continue.) An instructor should be part of the messenger's group (primarily for liability protection).
   b. Send an accident report form with the messengers.
   c. Send a map with the accident location marked on it.
   d. Put all requests and information that is sent out in written form. The spoken word can be easily miscommunicated (especially in an emergency) and written words allow for less interpretation. Ideally, there should be two copies: one copy should stay with the group, and one copy should go with the messengers.
   e. What is the notification priority?
      (1) Medical/rescue help will usually be contacted first.
      (2) Trip sponsors (the instructor's supervisor) can contact relatives, news media, etc.
   f. What contingency plans have been made?

B. **Evacuation Procedures**
   1. **Evacuation options**
      a. Patient walks out.
      b. Patient is carried out by group participants.
      c. Patient is carried out by rescue group (i.e., rangers, rescue squad, etc.)
      d. Patient is evacuated by helicopter or other mechanical means.
   2. **Evacuation considerations**
      a. Time
      b. Distance
      c. Terrain
      d. Weather

    e.   Condition of the patient

    f.   Cost

    g.   Mental and physical condition of the group

C. **Post-Incident Considerations**

    1.   The post incident report

    2.   Refund policy for the patient

    3.   Returning personal clothing and equipment

    4.   Recommended actions based on the incident

    5.   Implementation of recommendations

    6.   Dealing with the news media

    7.   Group dynamics

        a.   What has been the impact of the incident on the group?

        b.   How should the group be handled?

IV. **INSTRUCTIONAL STRATEGIES & MATERIALS:**

A. **Timing**

This lesson should be taught to WEA students before they go on any small group overnights without staff, or by the end of the second week.

B. **Activities**

This lesson is usually presented in a lecture/discussion format. It can also use role playing with a simulated accident.

C. **Materials**

Accident report form

40. Risk Management and Safety

I. **GOAL**: To have participants understand what a "Risk Management Plan" is, understand the considerations in pre-trip planning, and assemble a first aid kit.

II. **OBJECTIVES**:
A. Participants will be able to define "Risk Management Plan" and list considerations in the development of the plan.
B. Participants will be able to list pre-trip considerations in emergency planning.
C. Participants will be able to assemble a first aid kit and explain the purpose of each item in the kit.
D. Participants will be able to explain what training is necessary for wilderness leaders.

III. **CONTENT**:
A. **Risk Management Plan**
1. **Definition**: "...a systematic plan for reducing injuries...instituted through the policy board of the agency and implemented throughout the organization" (van der Smissen, 1980).
2. **Risk Management Plan aspects** (van der Smissen, 1980). An emergency procedure for accidents should include:
a. An accident form – *Pass around a sample form and discuss it.*
b. First aid training – *Discuss different types*:
(1) Standard First Aid, Emergency Medical Technician, Wilderness First Responder, Wilderness Emergency Medical Technician, etc.
(2) Cardio-Pulmonary Resuscitation
(3) Basic Water Rescue, Advanced Life Saving, Water Safety Instructorship, etc.

© 1992
The Wilderness Education Association
P.O. Box 89
Saranac Lake, New York 12983
(518) 891-2915 ext. 254

3. **A plan for supervision**
    a. **General** – Someone supervises participants within a given activity or area (e.g., campground supervisor).
    b. **Specific** – Someone is directly involved with participants in the activity (e.g., rockclimbing instructor).
4. **Safety rules, regulations, and procedures, and the need for an attitude of safety** should be emphasized.
5. **Inservice training should include the following topics:**
    a. **Capabilities of participants** – Recognize the physical condition and limitations of participants.
    b. **First aid and emergency procedures**
    c. **Safety awareness and safety procedures for activities**
    d. **How to supervise**
        (1) Be able to identify dangerous conditions.
        (2) Anticipate dangerous and potentially dangerous situations.
        (3) Teach appropriate safety procedures and practices and insure that participants adhere to these practices.
        (4) A leader should communicate the physical and technical risk involved in the activity to the participant.
6. **Technical skills as required**
    a. Regular inspection and maintenance of facilities and equipment.
    b. Programs based on:
        (1) Progression of activities in relation to developmental ability, skill and experience.
        (2) Qualified leadership and proper equipment.
        (3) Appropriate safety and instructional practices.
7. **A public relations program** which may include accident insurance for program participants.
8. **Working with the program insurance broker and lawyer,** educating them about the activities, safety procedures, and policies of the program.
    (van der Smissen, 1980).

9. The importance of tracking near misses (close calls)

    a. Near misses are occurrences that result in little or no injury or damage.

    b. It is important to track near misses to identify situations and patterns that may potentially lead to accidents.

B. **Pre-Trip Considerations**

1. **Medical histories and physicals**
   Leaders must be familiar with participants' medical histories and, if deemed appropriate, physicals may be required of participants. *This may be an appropriate time to discuss medical histories within the group. It might be mentioned that this information is usually available only to the leaders but, since in WEA courses everyone is a potential leader, medical histories are shared with everyone. Medical experiences, although sometimes embarrassing, are of great educational value.*

2. **Equipment maintenance**
   Stoves, ropes, tents, and vehicles must be in proper working order.

3. **Environmental considerations**
   Proper precautions must be taken concerning:
       a. Weather
       b. Terrain
       c. Animals, insects, and plants

4. **First aid kit**
       a. Is there an up-to-date and complete first aid kit? *Review the group's first aid kit at this time and explain the purpose and use of each item.*
       b. Does everyone who is qualified to use the first aid kit know where it is?

5. **Emergency and evacuation procedures**
   These should be developed before the trip and are discussed in greater detail in the "Emergency Procedures" lesson.

6. **Emergency contacts**
       a. Rescue/management personnel
       b. Group sponsors
       c. Relatives of each participant.

d.   Individuals familiar with the area of the expedition so that individuals in the group can be contacted in case of an outside emergency. This may include local rangers, staff, former staff, or former participants.

            At this time, the instructor can share telephone numbers of local personnel in the event of an emergency on the course.

7. **Evacuation routes**
    a.   Evacuation routes should be considered for each portion of the course.
    b.   How and where can you evacuate to?
    c.   Where is the nearest telephone?

IV. INSTRUCTIONAL STRATEGIES & MATERIALS:

A. **Timing**

This lesson should be taught to WEA students before they go on any small group overnights without staff, or by the end of the second week.

B. **Activities**

This lesson is usually presented in a lecture/discussion format. It can also use role playing with a simulated accident.

C. **Materials**
1.   First aid kit
2.   Accident report form

References

Chapter 1   Bathing and Washing

Petzoldt, P. (1984). *The new wilderness handbook* (2nd ed.). New York: W. W. Norton & Company. (Original work published in 1974)

Simer, P., & Sullivan, J. (1983). *The National Outdoor Leadership School's wilderness guide*. New York: Simon and Schuster.

Vivian, E. (1973). *Sourcebook for environmental education*. St.Louis: C. V. Mosby.

Chapter 2   Campsite Selection

Hart, J. (1977). *Walking softly in the wilderness*. San Francisco: Sierra Club Books.

Peacock, D. (1990, October). A practical guide to grizzly country. *Backpacker*, 18 (6), 80-85.

Petzoldt, P. (1984). *The new wilderness handbook* (2nd ed.). New York: W. W. Norton & Company. (Original work published in 1974)

Simer, P., & Sullivan, J. (1983). *The National Outdoor Leadership School's wilderness guide*. New York: Simon and Schuster.

Wilderness Education Association. *Instructors manual* [Manual]. Unpublished.

Chapter 3   Clothing Selection

Denner, J. C. (1990). *A primer on clothing systems for cold-weather field work* (Open-File Report 89-415). U.S. Department of the Interior. Bow, NH: U.S. Geological Survey.

Forgey, W. W. (1985). *Hypothermia: Death by exposure*. Merrillville, IN: ICS Books, Inc.

Hart, J. (1977). *Walking softly in the wilderness*. San Francisco: Sierra Club Books.

Petzoldt, P. (1984). *The new wilderness handbook* (2nd ed.). New York: W. W. Norton & Company. (Original work published in 1974)

Simer, P., & Sullivan, J. (1983). *The National Outdoor Leadership School's wilderness guide*. New York: Simon and Schuster.

Chapter 4   Decision Making

Buell, L. (1983). *Outdoor leadership competency: A manual for self-assessment and staff evaluation*. Greenfield, MA: Environmental Awareness Publications.

Cockrell, D. (Ed.). (1991). *The wilderness educator: The Wilderness Education Association curriculum guide*. Merrillville, IN: ICS Books, Inc.

Hersey, P., & Blanchard, K. H. (1982). *Management of organizational behavior: Utilizing human resources* (4th ed.). Englewood, NJ: Prentice-Hall, Inc.

Petzoldt, P. (1984). *The new wilderness handbook* (2nd ed.). New York: W. W. Norton & Company. (Original work published in 1974)

Sessoms, H. D., & Stevenson, J. L. (1981). *Leadership and group dynamics in recreation services*. Boston: Allyn and Bacon, Inc.

Weiss, R. (1987, July 25). How dare we?: Scientists seek the sources of risk-taking behavior. *Science News, 132* (4), 57-59.

Chapter 5   Environmental Ethics and Backcountry Conservation Practices

Cockrell, D. (Ed.). (1991). *The wilderness educator: The Wilderness Education Association curriculum guide*. Merrillville, IN: ICS Books, Inc.

Leopold, A. (1966). *A Sand County almanac: With essays on conservation from Round River*. New York: Ballantine Books.

Wilderness Education Association. (1989). *The WEA affiliate handbook: For current and prospective affiliate members*. Saranac Lake, NY: Wilderness Education Association.

Chapter 6   Expedition Behavior

Johnson, D. W., & Johnson, F. (1987). *Joining together: Group theory and group skills* (3rd ed.). Englewood Cliffs, NJ: Prentice-Hall, Inc.

Petzoldt, P. (1984). *The new wilderness handbook* (2nd ed.). New York: W. W. Norton & Company. (Original work published in 1974)

Chapter 7   Fire Site Preparation and Care

Boy Scouts of America. (1984). *Fieldbook* (3rd ed.). Irving, TX: Boy Scouts of America. (Original work published in 1944)

Cole, D. N. (1986). *NOLS Conservation Practices*. Lander, WY: Author.

Hammitt, W. E., & Cole, D. N. (1987). *Wildland recreation: Ecology and management* (p. 34). New York: John Wiley & Sons.

Hampton, B., & Cole, D. (1988). *Soft paths*. Harrisburg, PA: Stackpole Books.

Jacobson, C. (1986). *The new wilderness canoeing & camping*. Merrillville, IN: ICS Books, Inc.

Mason, B. S. (1939). *Woodcraft*. New York: A. S. Barnes & Company.

Petzoldt, P. (1984). *The new wilderness handbook* (2nd ed.). New York: W. W. Norton & Company. (Original work published in 1974)

Phillips, J. (1986). *Campground cookery: Outdoor living skills series* [Instructor manual] (2nd ed.). Jefferson City, MO: Missouri Department of Conservation. (Original work published in 1983)

Simer, P., & Sullivan, J. (1983). *The National Outdoor Leadership School's wilderness guide*. New York: Simon and Schuster.

Chapter 8   Fire Building

Boy Scouts of America. (1984). *Fieldbook* (3rd ed.). Irving, TX: Boy Scouts of America. (Original work published in 1944)

Petzoldt, P. (1984). *The new wilderness handbook* (2nd ed.). New York: W. W. Norton & Company. (Original work published in 1974)

Simer, P., & Sullivan, J. (1983). *The National Outdoor Leadership School's wilderness guide*. New York: Simon and Schuster.

Chapter 9   Group Processing and Debriefing

Quinsland, L. K., & Van Ginkel, A. (1984). How to process experience. *Journal of Experiential Education*, 7 (2), 8-13.

Chapter 10   Group Development

Caple, R. B. (1978, November). The sequential stages of group development. *Small Group Behavior*, 9 (3), 470-476.

Johnson, D. W., & Johnson, F. (1987). *Joining together: Group theory and group skills* (3rd ed.). Englewood Cliffs, NJ: Prentice-Hall, Inc.

Jones, J. E. (1973). A model of group development. In Jones, J. E., & Pfeiffer, J. W. (Eds.). *The annual handbook for group facilitators*. LaJolla, CA: University Associates, p. 129.

Kalisch, K. (1979). *The role of the instructor in the Outward Bound process*. Three Lakes, WI: Wheaton College.

Schoel, J., Prouty, D., & Radcliffe, P. (1988). *Islands of healing: A guide to adventure based counseling*. Hamilton, MA: Project Adventure, Inc.

Shaw, M. (1981). *Group dynamics: The psychology of small group behavior* (3rd ed.). New York: McGraw-Hill Books.

Chapter 11   Latrine Construction and Use

Hart, J. (1977). *Walking softly in the wilderness*. San Francisco: Sierra Club Books.

Meyer, K. (1989). *How to shit in the woods*. Berkeley, CA: Ten Speed Press.

Simer, P., & Sullivan, J. (1983). *The National Outdoor Leadership School's wilderness guide*. New York: Simon and Schuster.

Chapter 12   Leadership

Buell, L. (1983). *Outdoor leadership competency: A manual for self-assessment and staff evaluation*. Greenfield, MA: Environmental Awareness Publications.

Clark K. E., & Clark, M. B. (1990). *Measures of leadership*. West Orange, NJ: Leadership Library of America.

Petzoldt, P. (1984). *The new wilderness handbook* (2nd ed.). New York: W. W. Norton & Company. (Original work published in 1974)

Rosenbach, W. E., & Taylor, R. L. (Eds.). *Contemporary issues in leadership*. Boulder, CO: Westview Press.

Chapter 13   Nutrition and Rations Planning

Drury, J. K. (1986, Fall). Idea notebook: Wilderness food planning in the computer age. *Journal of Experiential Education*, 9, (3) 36-40.

Petzoldt, P. (1984). *The new wilderness handbook* (2nd ed.). New York: W. W. Norton & Company. (Original work published in 1974)

Richard, S., Orr, D., & Lindholm, C. (Ed.). (1988). *The NOLS cookery: Experience the art of outdoor cooking* (2nd ed.). Lander, WY: National Outdoor Leadership School.

Simer, P., & Sullivan, J. (1983). *The National Outdoor Leadership School's wilderness guide*. New York: Simon and Schuster.

Chapter 14   Pack Adjustments

Petzoldt, P. (1984). *The new wilderness handbook* (2nd ed.). New York: W. W. Norton & Company. (Original work published in 1974)

Simer, P., & Sullivan, J. (1983). *The National Outdoor Leadership School's wilderness guide*. New York: Simon and Schuster.

Chapter 15   Pack Packing

Petzoldt, P. (1984). *The new wilderness handbook* (2nd ed.). New York: W. W. Norton & Company. (Original work published in 1974)

Simer, P., & Sullivan, J. (1983). *The National Outdoor Leadership School's wilderness guide*. New York: Simon and Schuster.

Chapter 16   Personal Hygiene

Petzoldt, P. (1984). *The new wilderness handbook* (2nd ed.). New York: W. W. Norton & Company. (Original work published in 1974)

Chapter 17   Stove Operation

Hart, J. (1977). *Walking softly in the wilderness*. San Francisco: Sierra Club Books.

Simer, P., & Sullivan, J. (1983). *The National Outdoor Leadership School's wilderness guide*. New York: Simon and Schuster.

Chapter 18   Teaching Technique

Petzoldt, P. (1984). *The new wilderness handbook* (2nd ed.). New York: W. W. Norton & Company. (Original work published in 1974)

Chapter 19   Trail Technique: Introductory

Petzoldt, P. (1984). *The new wilderness handbook* (2nd ed.). New York: W. W. Norton & Company. (Original work published in 1974)

Simer, P., & Sullivan, J. (1983). *The National Outdoor Leadership School's wilderness guide*. New York: Simon and Schuster.

Chapter 20   Trail Technique: Advanced

Hart, J. (1977). *Walking softly in the wilderness*. San Francisco: Sierra Club Books.

Petzoldt, P. (1984). *The new wilderness handbook* (2nd ed.). New York: W. W. Norton & Company. (Original work published in 1974)

Simer, P., & Sullivan, J. (1983). *The National Outdoor Leadership School's wilderness guide.* New York: Simon and Schuster.

Chapter 21   Trip Planning

Wilderness Recreation Leadership Program. (1984). *Winter practicum manual.* [Manual] Saranac Lake, NY: North Country Community College.

Wilderness Recreation Leadership Program. (1985). *Winter practicum manual.* [Manual] Saranac Lake, NY: North Country Community College.

Wilderness Recreation Leadership Program. (1986). *Winter practicum manual.* [Manual] Saranac Lake, NY: North Country Community College.

Chapter 22   Water Safety

American National Red Cross (1977). *Canoeing.* Garden City, NY: Doubleday & Company, Inc.

American Red Cross (1979). *Lifesaving: Rescue and safety.* Garden City, NY: Doubleday & Company, Inc.

Forgey, W. W. (1985). *Hypothermia: Death by exposure.* Merrillville, IN: ICS Books, Inc.

Priest, S., & Dixon, T. (1990). *Safety practices in adventure programming.* Boulder, CO: Association of Experiential Education.

Chapter 23   Water Treatment

Backer, H. (1989). Field water disinfection. In Auerbach & Geehr (Eds.), *Management of wilderness and environmental emergencies.* St. Louis: C.V. Mosby.

Kahn, F. H., & Visscher, B. R. (1977, April-May). Water disinfection in the wilderness: A simple method of iodination. *Summit* , 23 (3), 11-14.

Schimelpfenig, T., & Lindsey, L. (1991). *NOLS wilderness first aid.* Lander, WY: National Outdoor Leadership School.

Chapter 24   WEA History

Cockrell, D. (Ed.). (1991). *The wilderness educator: The Wilderness Education Association curriculum guide.* Merrillville, IN: ICS Books, Inc.

National Outdoor Leadership School (1987). *State of the school* [Annual report]. Lander, WY: Author.

National Outdoor Leadership School (1991). *National Outdoor Leadership School 1991 catalog of courses.* Lander, WY: Author.

Outward Bound (1987). *Instructor's field manual: North Carolina Outward Bound School.* Morganton, NC: North Carolina Outward Bound School.

Wilderness Education Association. (1989). *The WEA affiliate handbook: For current and prospective affiliate members.* Saranac Lake, NY: Wilderness Education Association.

Chapter 25 Weather

Boy Scouts of America. (1984). *Fieldbook* (3rd ed.). Irving, TX: Boy Scouts of America. (Original work published in 1944)

Fisher, R. M. (1955). *Talk about the weather.* New York: Birk & Co., Inc.

Hardy, R., Wright, P., Kington, J., & Gribbin, J. (1982). *The weather book.* Boston: Little, Brown and Company.

Kovachick, R. J. (Ed.) (n.d.). *United States weather: Northeastern New York and New England edition* (pp. 27-29). Albany, NY: WTEN10 and WCDC 19.

Lehr, P. E., Burnett, R. W., & Zim, H. S. (1964). *Weather: A guide to phenomena and forecasts* (16-20, 142-145). New York: Golden Press.

Petterssen, S. (1958). *Introduction to meteorology* (2nd ed.). New York: McGraw Hill-Books.

Simer, P., & Sullivan, J. (1983). *The National Outdoor Leadership School's wilderness guide.* New York: Simon and Schuster.

Spooner, T. (1944). *Man's heritage of the skies: The ways of weather and climate and how they reach into our daily lives.* (p. 9). Pittsburgh: Westinghouse Electric & Manufacturing Company.

United States Weather Bureau. (1962). *Cloud forms* [poster].

Chapter 26 Food Identification

Drury, J. K. (1986, Fall). Idea notebook: Wilderness food planning in the computer age. *Journal of Experiential Education, 9,* (3) 36-40.

Petzoldt, P. (1984). *The new wilderness handbook* (2nd ed.). New York: W. W. Norton & Company. (Original work published in 1974)

Simer, P., & Sullivan, J. (1983). *The National Outdoor Leadership School's wilderness guide.* New York: Simon and Schuster.

Chapter 27 Food Protection

Boy Scouts of America. (1984). *Fieldbook* (3rd ed.). Irving, TX: Boy Scouts of America. (Original work published in 1944)

Chapter 28 Food Waste Disposal

Petzoldt, P. (1984). *The new wilderness handbook* (2nd ed.). New York: W. W. Norton & Company. (Original work published in 1974)

Simer, P., & Sullivan, J. (1983). *The National Outdoor Leadership School's wilderness guide.* New York: Simon and Schuster.

Chapter 29 Frying and Baking

Petzoldt, P. (1984). *The new wilderness handbook* (2nd ed.). New York: W. W. Norton & Company. (Original work published in 1974)

Richard, S., Orr, D., & Lindholm, C. (Ed.). (1988). *The NOLS cookery: Experience the art of outdoor cooking* (2nd ed.). Lander, WY: National Outdoor Leadership School.

Simer, P., & Sullivan, J. (1983). *The National Outdoor Leadership School's wilderness guide.* New York: Simon and Schuster.

Chapter 30   Granola Preparation
Petzoldt, P. (1984). *The new wilderness handbook* (2nd ed.). New York: W. W. Norton & Company. (Original work published in 1974)

Richard, S., Orr, D., & Lindholm, C. (Ed.). (1988). *The NOLS cookery: Experience the art of outdoor cooking* (2nd ed.). Lander, WY: National Outdoor Leadership School.

Simer, P., & Sullivan, J. (1983). *The National Outdoor Leadership School's wilderness guide.* New York: Simon and Schuster.

Chapter 31   Introductory Cooking
Petzoldt, P. (1984). *The new wilderness handbook* (2nd ed.). New York: W. W. Norton & Company. (Original work published in 1974)

Richard, S., Orr, D., & Lindholm, C. (Ed.). (1988). *The NOLS cookery: Experience the art of outdoor cooking* (2nd ed.). Lander, WY: National Outdoor Leadership School.

Simer, P., & Sullivan, J. (1983). *The National Outdoor Leadership School's wilderness guide.* New York: Simon and Schuster.

Chapter 32   Yeast Baking
Richard, S., Orr, D., & Lindholm, C. (Ed.). (1988). *The NOLS cookery: Experience the art of outdoor cooking* (2nd ed.). Lander, WY: National Outdoor Leadership School.

Chapter 34   Map Interpretation
Braasch, G. (1973, Fall). Reading a map at a glance. *Backpacker,* p. 34.

Jacobson, C. (1988). *The basic essentials of map & compass.* Merrillville, IN: ICS Books, Inc.

Kjellstrom, B. (1976). *Be expert with map and compass: The orienteering handbook.* New York: Charles Scribner's Sons.

Chapter 35   Compass: An Introduction
Kjellstrom, B. (1976). *Be expert with map and compass: The orienteering handbook.* New York: Charles Scribner's Sons.

Warren, J. W. (1986, May). Map and compass fundamentals. *Adirondac,* L (4), 12-16.

Chapter 36   Combining the Map and Compass
Kjellstrom, B. (1976). *Be expert with map and compass: The orienteering handbook.* New York: Charles Scribner's Sons.

Warren, J. W. (1986, May). Map and compass fundamentals. *Adirondac,* L (4), 12-16.

Chapter 37   Route Finding with Map and Compass

Kjellstrom, B. (1976). *Be expert with map and compass: The orienteering handbook.* New York: Charles Scribner's Sons.

Warren, J. W. (1986, May). Map and compass fundamentals. *Adirondac,* L (4), 12-16.

Chapter 38   Triangulation with Map and Compass

Kjellstrom, B. (1976). *Be expert with map and compass: The orienteering handbook.* New York: Charles Scribner's Sons.

Chapter 39   Emergency Procedures

Johanson, K. M. (Ed.). (1984). *Accepted peer practices in adventure programming.* Boulder, CO: Association for Experiential Education.

van der Smissen, B. J. (1980). *Legal liability: Adventure activities.* Las Cruces, NM: Educational Resources Information Center.

Chapter 40   Risk Management and Safety

Johanson, K. M. (Ed.). (1984). *Accepted peer practices in adventure programming.* Boulder, CO: Association for Experiential Education.

van der Smissen, B. J. (1980). *Legal liability: Adventure activities.* Las Cruces, NM: Educational Resources Information Center.

Bibliography

American National Red Cross (1977). *Canoeing.* Garden City, NY: Doubleday & Company, Inc.

American Red Cross (1979). *Lifesaving: Rescue and safety.* Garden City, NY: Doubleday & Company, Inc.

Backer, H. (1989). Field water disinfection. In Auerbach & Geehr (Eds.), *Management of wilderness and environmental emergencies.* St. Louis: C.V. Mosby.

Bloch, J. D., & Patzkowsky, G. L. (1985, January). Giardiasis. *Family Practice Recertification, 7* (1), 106-119, 122.

Boy Scouts of America. (1980). *Lifesaving.* Irving, TX: Boy Scouts of America.

Boy Scouts of America. (1984). *Fieldbook* (3rd ed.). Irving, TX: Boy Scouts of America. (Original work published in 1944)

Boy Scouts of America. (1989). *Canoeing.* Irving, TX: Boy Scouts of America.

Braasch, G. (1973, Fall). Reading a map at a glance. *Backpacker,* p. 34.

Buell, L. (1983). *Outdoor leadership competency: A manual for self-assessment and staff evaluation.* Greenfield, MA: Environmental Awareness Publications.

Caple, R. B. (1978, November). The sequential stages of group development. *Small Group Behavior, 9* (3), 470-476.

Clark K. E., & Clark, M. B. (1990). *Measures of leadership.* West Orange, NJ: Leadership Library of America.

Cockrell, D. (Ed.). (1991). *The wilderness educator: The Wilderness Education Association curriculum guide.* Merrillville, IN: ICS Books, Inc.

Cole, D. N. (1986). *NOLS Conservation Practices.* Lander, WY: The National Outdoor Leadership School.

Denner, J. C. (1990). *A primer on clothing systems for cold-weather field work* (Open-File Report 89-415). U.S. Department of the Interior. Bow, NH: U.S. Geological Survey.

Drury, J. K. (1986, Fall). Idea notebook: Wilderness food planning in the computer age. *Journal of Experiential Education, 9,* (3) 36-40.

Ferris, M. (1986, August). Update on giardiasis. *Adirondac, L* (7) pp. 26-27.

Fisher, R. M. (1955). *Talk about the weather.* New York: Birk & Co., Inc.

Forgey, W. W. (1985). *Hypothermia: Death by exposure.* Merrillville, IN: ICS Books, Inc.

© 1992
The Wilderness Education Association
P.O. Box 89
Saranac Lake, New York 12983
(518) 891-2915 ext. 254

Forgey, W. W. (1987). *Wilderness medicine.* Merrillville, IN: ICS Books, Inc.

Gormley, C. (1979). *Group backpacking: A leader's manual.* South Plainfield, NJ: Group Work Today.

Hammitt, W. E., & Cole, D. N. (1987). *Wildland recreation: Ecology and management* (p. 34). New York: John Wiley & Sons.

Hampton, B., & Cole, D. (1988). *Soft paths.* Harrisburg, PA: Stackpole Books.

Hardy, R., Wright, P., Kington, J., & Gribbin, J. (1982). *The weather book.* Boston: Little, Brown and Company.

Hart, J. (1977). *Walking softly in the wilderness.* San Francisco: Sierra Club Books.

Hersey, P., & Blanchard, K. H. (1982). *Management of organizational behavior: Utilizing human resources* (4th ed.). Englewood, NJ: Prentice-Hall, Inc.

Jacobson, C. (1986). *The new wilderness canoeing & camping.* Merrillville, IN: ICS Books, Inc.

Jacobson, C. (1988). *The basic essentials of map & compass.* Merrillville, IN: ICS Books, Inc.

Johanson, K. M. (Ed.). (1984). *Accepted peer practices in adventure programming.* Boulder, CO: Association for Experiential Education.

Johnson, D. W., & Johnson, F. (1987). *Joining together: Group theory and group skills* (3rd ed.). Englewood Cliffs, NJ: Prentice-Hall, Inc.

Jones, J. E. (1973). A model of group development. In Jones, J. E., & Pfeiffer, J. W. (Eds.). *The annual handbook for group facilitators.* LaJolla, CA: University Associates, p. 129.

Kahn, F. H., & Visscher, B. R. (1977, April-May). Water disinfection in the wilderness: A simple method of iodination. *Summit,* 23 (3), 11-14.

Kalisch, K. (1979). *The role of the instructor in the Outward Bound process.* Three Lakes, WI: Wheaton College.

Kjellstrom, B. (1976). *Be expert with map and compass: The orienteering handbook.* New York: Charles Scribner's Sons.

Kovachick, R. J. (Ed.). (n.d.). *United States weather: Northeastern New York and New England edition* (pp. 27-29). Albany, NY: WTEN10 and WCDC 19.

Lappe, F. (1975). *Diet for a small planet.* New York: Ballantine Books.

Lehr, P. E., Burnett, R. W., & Zim, H. S. (1964). *Weather: A guide to phenomena and forecasts* (16-20, 142-145). New York: Golden Press.

Leopold, A. (1966). *A Sand County almanac: With essays on conservation from Round River.* New York: Ballantine Books.

Mason, B. S. (1939). *Woodcraft.* New York: A. S. Barnes & Company.

Meyer, K. (1989). *How to shit in the woods.* Berkeley, CA: Ten Speed Press.

National Outdoor Leadership School (1987). *State of the school* [Annual report]. Lander, WY: Author.

National Outdoor Leadership School (1991). *National Outdoor Leadership School 1991 catalog of courses.* Lander, WY: Author.

Outward Bound (1987). *Instructor's field manual: North Carolina Outward Bound School.* Morganton, NC: North Carolina Outward Bound School.

Outward Bound (1987). *Outward Bound USA: 25 years of service* [Annual report]. Greenwich, CT: Outward Bound USA.

Peacock, D. (1990, October). A practical guide to grizzly country. *Backpacker*, 18 (6), 80-85.

Petterssen, S. (1958). *Introduction to meteorology* (2nd ed.). New York: McGraw Hill-Books.

Petzoldt, P. (1984). *The new wilderness handbook* (2nd ed.). New York: W.W. Norton & Company. (Original work published in 1974)

Phillips, J. (1986). *Campground cookery: Outdoor living skills series* [Instructor manual] (2nd ed.). Jefferson City, MO: Missouri Department of Conservation. (Original work published in 1983)

Priest, S., & Dixon, T. (1990). *Safety practices in adventure programming*. Boulder, CO: Association of Experiential Education.

Quinsland, L. K., & Van Ginkel, A. (1984). How to process experience. *Journal of Experiential Education, 7* (2), 8-13.

Reifsnyder, W. E. (1980). *Weathering the wilderness: The Sierra Club guide to practical meteorology*. San Francisco: Sierra Club Books.

Richard, S., Orr, D., & Lindholm, C. (Ed.). (1988). *The NOLS cookery: Experience the art of outdoor cooking* (2nd ed.). Lander, WY: National Outdoor Leadership School.

Rosenbach, W. E., & Taylor, R. L. (Eds.). *Contemporary issues in leadership*. Boulder, CO: Westview Press.

Schimelpfenig, T., & Lindsey, L. (1991). *NOLS wilderness first aid*. Lander, WY: National Outdoor Leadership School.

Schoel, J., Prouty, D., & Radcliffe, P. (1988). *Islands of healing: A guide to adventure based counseling*. Hamilton, MA: Project Adventure, Inc.

Sessoms, H. D., & Stevenson, J. L. (1981). *Leadership and group dynamics in recreation services*. Boston: Allyn and Bacon, Inc.

Shaw, M. (1981). *Group dynamics: The psychology of small group behavior* (3rd ed.). New York: McGraw-Hill Books.

Simer, P., & Sullivan, J. (1983). *The National Outdoor Leadership School's wilderness guide*. New York: Simon and Schuster.

Spooner, T. (1944). *Man's heritage of the skies: The ways of weather and climate and how they reach into our daily lives* (p. 9). Pittsburgh: Westinghouse Electric & Manufacturing Company.

United States Weather Bureau. (1962). *Cloud forms* [poster].

van der Smissen, B. J. (1980). *Legal liability: Adventure activities*. Las Cruces, NM: Educational Resources Information Center.

Vivian, E. (1973). *Sourcebook for environmental education*. St. Louis: C.V. Mosby.

Warren, J. W. (1986, May). Map and compass fundamentals. *Adirondac*, L (4), 12-16.

Weiss, R. (1987, July 25). How dare we?: Scientists seek the sources of risk-taking behavior. *Science News, 132* (4), 57-59.

Welch, T. R. (1986, September 30). [Letter to the editor]. Unpublished letter. *Adirondac*.

Wilderness Education Association. *Instructors manual* [Manual]. Unpublished.

Wilderness Education Association. (1989). *The WEA affiliate handbook: For current and prospective affiliate members.* Saranac Lake, NY: Wilderness Education Association.

Wilderness Recreation Leadership Program. (1984). *Winter practicum manual.* [Manual] Saranac Lake, NY: North Country Community College.

Wilderness Recreation Leadership Program. (1985). *Winter practicum manual.* [Manual] Saranac Lake, NY: North Country Community College.

Wilderness Recreation Leadership Program. (1986). *Winter practicum manual.* [Manual] Saranac Lake, NY: North Country Community College.

Index

About the authors

Bruce Bonney has been teaching public high school social studies at Morrisville-Eaton Central School in Morrisville, New York for the past 22 years. A WEA instructor, Bruce is also owner and operator of Wilderness Education Services which contracts with public schools for wilderness education training. Bruce received his B.A. from Colgate University and his M.S. in history from Syracuse University. He is also an adjunct professor for North Country Community College.

Jack Drury is Associate Professor and Director of Wilderness Recreation Leadership at North Country Community College, a unit of the State University of New York (SUNY) in Saranac Lake, New York. He is a WEA instructor having taught WEA NSP courses annually since 1979. He is currently president of the Wilderness Education Association and holds a B.S. in recreation education from SUNY Cortland and a M.S. in education administration from SUNY, Plattsburgh.

Wilderness Education Association
Membership Application

PLEASE PRINT   [ ] New Member   [ ] Renewal   [ ] Address Change

Name _____

Address _____

City _____ State _____ Zip _____

Phone _____ Birth Date _____

Permanent address and phone (if different from above):

_____

My check in the amount of $ _____ is enclosed for my membership category indicated below: ?

[ ] $15 Student (full time) School _____
[ ] $20 Senior Citizen
[ ] $30 Individual
[ ] $45 Family
[ ] $80 Organizational
[ ] $100 Sustaining

[ ] $250 Corporate
[ ] $500 Supporting
[ ] $1000 Life
[ ] $5000 Wilderness Steward

International Members: Please Add $5

Please make checks payable to:
Wilderness Education Association
20 Winona Ave., Box 89
Saranac Lake, NY 12983
(518) 891-2915 ext. 254

Are you a WEA alumni?   Y   N

Year of graduation _____ 19 _____

Affiliate _____

How did you hear about WEA?

_____

Benefits of Membership

- WEA membership card
- WEA decal (new members only)
- 10% discount on outdoor equipment at *Indiana Camp Supply*
- 10% discount on *SOLO* wilderness medicine courses
- Subscription to quarterly newsletter
- WEA job referral service

NEW SUSTAINING, SUPPORTING, CORPORATE, LIFE AND WILDERNESS STEWARD MEMBERS WILL RECEIVE THESE ADDITIONAL BENEFITS:

- an autographed copy of Paul Petzoldt's *New Wilderness Handbook*
- a print of an original photograph by Robert Lindholm, a recipient of the Sierra Club's Ansel Adams Award

[ ] PLEASE APPLY ALL OF MY DUES TO THE GOOD WORK OF WEA. I WOULD RATHER NOT RECEIVE THESE ADDITIONAL BENEFITS.

A less tangible benefit is the satisfaction one receives from supporting our national effort.

THE WILDERNESS EDUCATION ASSOCIATION...

...is a non-profit membership organization that promotes wilderness education and preservation through wilderness leadership training at the college level. Affiliate organizations are accredited to offer WEA's National Standard Program for Outdoor Leadership Certification (NSP). Successful graduates of these programs receive WEA certification.

The WEA trains leaders, people who will have the good judgment and decision-making skills necessary to lead safe and environmentally-sound adventures. The WEA affiliate is not limited to teaching outdoor skills or providing challenging adventures. WEA program providers teach students to know their own abilities and limitations, to make quality judgment decisions, and to refrain from accepting responsibilities beyond their capabilities.

WEA MISSION STATEMENT

The purpose of the Wilderness Education Association is to promote the professionalization of outdoor leadership and thereby improve the quality and safety of outdoor trips and enhance the conservation of the wild outdoors.

WEA'S APPROACH

WEA promotes professionalism through several equally important strategies:
Certification and Affiliation • Membership and Development
Program Consultancy • Research

BENEFITS OF MEMBERSHIP

WEA membership card and decal
Discount on outdoor equipment and wilderness medicine courses
Subscription to quarterly newsletter
Wilderness job referral service

For further information concerning course content, current affiliated programs, course dates and locations, or membership information, write or call our national office:

Wilderness Education Association
20 Winona Avenue, Box 89
Saranac Lake, New York 12983
(518) 891-2915 ext. 254

You can help support the mission of the Wilderness Education Association by purchasing WEA resale items. Proceeds are used to develop, administer, and improve WEA programs. The WEA is training the leaders of tomorrow and appreciates your support to accomplish this important mission.

Other Titles by the Publisher:

THE WILDERNESS EDUCATOR: The WEA Curriculum Guide. Recommended as a supplement to *The Backcountry Classroom*, this is a textbook of outdoor adventure leadership principles and leadership evaluation techniques. $29.95

WILDERNESS MEDICINE, by Dr. William Forgey, M.D. Invaluable information for wilderness travelers. $7.95
CAMPFIRE STORIES: Things That Go Bump In The Night. 21 classic stories (each with an outline) that are easy to tell from memory. $9.95
WILDERNESS VISIONARIES. Profiles of six naturalists who made wilderness the central theme of their lives. It makes an important statement about the significance of wilderness in the evolution of North American culture. $9.95
THE BASIC ESSENTIAL SERIES for anyone interested in a refresher on outdoor skills. Each book provides the essential knowledge for a safe, enjoyable trip into the wilderness. $4.95 each. Titles include:
❑ Backpacking ❑ Camping ❑ Canoeing ❑ Cooking ❑ Cross-Country Skiing ❑ Desert Survival ❑ Edible Wild Plants ❑ Mountaineering ❑ First-Aid For The Outdoors ❑ Hypothermia ❑ Kayaking Whitewater ❑ Knots ❑ Map & Compass ❑ Minimizing Impact ❑ Mountain Biking ❑ Photography Outdoors ❑ Rafting ❑ Rescue From The Backcountry ❑ Rock Climbing ❑ Solo Canoeing ❑ Sea Kayaking ❑ Survival ❑ Women In The Outdoors

These books are available from:

WEA	ICS Books, Inc.
20 Winona Ave., Box 89	One Tower Plaza, 107 E. 89th Ave.
Saranac Lake, NY 12983	Merrillville, IN 46410
(518) 891-2915 ext. 254	(800) 541-7323

Also available from WEA:

WEA AFFILIATE HANDBOOK. An outline of the WEA curriculum, evaluation process, affiliation procedures, and course administration information. $13.50
NEW WILDERNESS HANDBOOK, by Paul Petzoldt, 2nd edition. $10.95
WEA WOOL BASEBALL CAPS. Green or Navy Blue. $10.95
WEA FIELD MUG. 12 oz. insulated mug imprinted with the WEA logo. $5.50
WEA T-SHIRT. WEA logo on 100% heavyweight cotton. Fuchsia, Jade, Navy Blue, Teal. Sizes M-XL. $10.95
WEA DECAL. 4-color logo sticker with white vinyl backing, 2.5" x 2.25". $1.50
WEA PATCH. 7-color WEA logo embroidered on a 3" hexagonal patch. $4.00